O O L

OXFORD ONCOLOGY LIBRARY

Renal Cancer

Edited by

Professor Tim Eisen

University of Cambridge
Department of Oncology
Addenbrooke's Hospital
Cambridge, UK

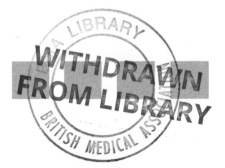

OXFORD
UNIVERSITY PRESS

OXFORD
UNIVERSITY PRESS

Great Clarendon Street, Oxford OX2 6DP

Oxford University Press is a department of the University of Oxford.
It furthers the University's objective of excellence in research, scholarship,
and education by publishing worldwide in

Oxford New York

Auckland Cape Town Dar es Salaam Hong Kong Karachi
Kuala Lumpur Madrid Melbourne Mexico City Nairobi
New Delhi Shanghai Taipei Toronto

With offices in

Argentina Austria Brazil Chile Czech Republic France Greece
Guatemala Hungary Italy Japan Poland Portugal Singapore
South Korea Switzerland Thailand Turkey Ukraine Vietnam

Oxford is a registered trade mark of Oxford University Press
in the UK and in certain other countries

Published in the United States
by Oxford University Press Inc., New York

© Oxford University Press, 2010

British Library Cataloguing in Publication Data

Data available

Library of Congress Cataloging in Publication Data

Data available

Typeset by Newgen Imaging Systems (P) Ltd, Chennai, India
Printed in Great Britain
on acid-free paper by
Ashford Colour Press Ltd., Gosport, Hampshire

ISBN 978–0–19–956231–2

10 9 8 7 6 5 4 3 2 1

Contents

Preface

The management of kidney cancer has developed enormously over the last decade. Advances in surgical techniques have recently been matched by a range of new drugs which target the tumour blood supply so crucial to the growth and spread of kidney cancer. With these advances have come new challenges for medical and nursing staff treating patients with kidney cancer. This book is a handy reference by international experts in the field. It covers the essential information needed to manage patients with kidney cancer in an easily accessible format. It will be of particular use to trainees in a number of medical, nursing and allied disciplines caring for patients with kidney cancer.

Abbreviations

3D	three-dimensional
5-FU	5-fluorouracil
AJCC	American Joint Committee on Cancer
AML	angiomyolipoma
BHD	Birt–Hogg–Dubé syndrome
CA IX	carbonic anhydrase IX
CCRC	clear cell renal carcinoma
CNS	central nervous system
CR	complete response
CT	computed tomography
DCs	dendritic cells
DFS	disease-free survival
DMSA	dimercaptosuccinic acid
ECOG	Eastern Cooperative Oncology Group
eGFR	estimation of glomerular filtration rate
EOTRC	European Organization for Research and Treatment of Cancer
FDA	Food and Drug Administration
FDG	fluorodeoxyglucose
Flt-3	foetal liver tyrosine kinase-3
Gp	glycoprotein
HFSR	hand–foot skin reaction
HIF	hypoxia-inducible factors
HL	hereditary leiomyomatosis
HLRCC	hereditary leiomyomatosis renal cell carcinoma
HSCT	hematopoietic stem cell transplantation
HSP	heat shock protein
IFN	interferon
IGA	image-guided ablation
IL-2	interleukin-2
IV	intravenous
IVC	inferior vena cava
MDRD	modification of diet in renal disease

MPR	multiplanar reformation
mRCC	metastatic renal cell carcinoma
MRC	Medical Research Council
MRI	magnetic resonance imaging
MSKCC	Memorial Sloan-Kettering Cancer Center
mTOR	mammalian target of rapamycin
NCCN	National Comprehensive Cancer Network
NCI	National Cancer Institute
NICE	National Institute for Health and Clinical Excellence
NK	natural killer (cells)
PD	progressive disease
PDGF	platelet-derived growth factor
PET	positron emission tomography
PFS	progression-free survival
PR	partial response
PRCC	papillary renal cell carcinoma
RCC	renal cell carcinoma
RECIST	response evaluation criteria in solid tumours
RFA	radiofrequency ablation
TAE	transarterial embolization
TARGET	The Treatment Approach in Renal Cancer Global Evaluation Trial
TBRR	tumour burden reduction rate
TGFα	transforming growth factor-α
TKIs	tyrosine kinase inhibitors
UISS	UCLA Integrated Staging System
VEGF	vascular endothelial growth factor
VHL	von Hippel–Lindau (disease)
WHO	World Health Organization

Contributors

David Breen
Southampton General Hospital
Southampton, UK

Tim Eisen
University of Cambridge
Department of Oncology
Addenbrooke's Hospital
Cambridge, UK

Khalid Enver
Southampton General Hospital
Southampton, UK

Bernard Escudier
Département de Médecine
Institut Gustave Roussy
Villejuif, France

Michael J. Fisch
Department of General Oncology
MD Anderson Cancer Center
Houston, Texas, USA

Karim Fizazi
Département de Médecine
Institut Gustave Roussy
Villejuif, France

Martin Gore
Royal Marsden Hospital
London, UK

Marine Gross Goupil
Département de Médecine
Institut Gustave Roussy
Villejuif, France

Sheeba Irshad
Medical Oncology Specialist Trainee
Royal Marsden Hospital
London, UK

Christophe Massard
Département de Médecine
Institut Gustave Roussy
Villejuif, France

Jessica Masterson
Division of Cancer Medicine, MD
Anderson Cancer Centre
Houston, Texas, USA

Arnaud Méjean
Department of Urology
Necker Hospital
Paris, France

Paul Nathan
Mount Vernon Cancer Centre
Northwood, UK

David Quinn
University of Southern
California
Los Angeles, California, USA

Aslam Sohaib
Department of Imaging
Royal Marsden Hospital
London, UK

Nizar M. Tannir
Department of Genitourinary
Medical Oncology
MD Anderson Cancer Center
Houston, Texas, USA

Marc-Olivier Timsit
Department of Urology
Necker Hospital
Paris, France

Maxine Tran
University of Cambridge
Department of Oncology
Addenbrooke's Hospital
Cambridge, UK

Anup Vinayan
Mount Vernon Cancer Centre
Northwood, UK

Chapter 1

Aetiology and molecular basis of disease

Maxine Tran and Tim Eisen

Key points

- Renal cancer is the commonest malignancy of the kidney
- Clear cell renal cancer is the commonest form of renal cancer
- Smoking accounts for 25% of the disease
- Different genetic abnormalities and molecular mechanisms underpin the different histological subtypes
- Defective function of the *VHL* gene underlies 80% of clear cell renal cancers.

Renal cell carcinoma (RCC) accounts for 2–3% of all adult cancers and is steadily increasing worldwide. It causes significant morbidity and mortality with over 6,600 patients being diagnosed in the United Kingdom every year, of which more than half will eventually succumb and die from the disease. Recent advances in our understanding of the aetiology and molecular basis of kidney cancer have directed the development of new treatment strategies, which have allowed entry into a new era in the management of patients with metastatic disease.

1.1 **Aetiology of disease**

Renal cancer is twice as common in males as in females and is most prevalent in the general population in the sixth decade of life. Large epidemiological studies have established risk factors for renal cancer that include cigarette smoking (most important risk factor accounting for over one-quarter of diseases), obesity, end-stage renal failure, western-style diet, hypertension, and a family history of renal cancer. Kidney cancer was once considered a single disease; however, it is now evident that there are a number of distinct subtypes, each with different histological and prognostic features, and each caused by mutations in different genes.

Table 1.1 The Heidelberg classification of adult renal epithelial neoplasms	
Benign tumours	**Malignant tumours**
Papillary renal adenoma	Conventional or clear cell renal cell carcinoma
Metanephric adenoma	Papillary renal cell carcinoma
Oncocytoma	Chromophobe renal cell carcinoma
	Collecting duct carcinoma (including renal medullary carcinoma)
	Renal cell carcinoma, unclassified

Several classification systems have been described for renal cancer. The popular Heidelberg classification is widely adopted and simply divides renal tumours into benign and malignant groups (Table 1.1). The World Health Organization (WHO) classification of kidney tumours was introduced in 2004 and provides a more comprehensive classification system (Table 1.2).

1.1.1 Benign renal epithelial tumours

Benign renal epithelial tumours include the following subtypes:

- Papillary renal adenomas
- Oncocytomas
- Metanephric renal adenomas.

1.1.1.1 *Papillary renal adenomas*

Papillary renal adenomas are very common lesions and are composed of basophilic cuboidal cells arranged in a typically tubulopapillary network. They tend to be multiple in nature and are usually diagnosed incidentally on nephrectomy specimens performed for other pathologies. Papillary renal adenomas are morphologically and histologically similar to low-grade papillary RCCs, the defining criteria being size, so that an adenoma characteristically is less than 5mm in diameter. It therefore follows that papillary renal adenomas have been postulated to be precursor lesions to papillary cell carcinomas.

1.1.1.2 *Renal oncocytomas*

Renal oncocytomas account for 5% of renal neoplasms in which eosinophilic round cells packed with numerous mitochondria, arranged in nests, are separated by hypocellular stroma.

1.1.1.3 *Metanephric renal adenomas*

Metanephric renal adenomas are rare benign lesions. Affected patients are usually diagnosed incidentally and may also have the unusual paraneoplastic feature of polycythaemia caused by the production of erythropoietin tumour cell.

Table 1.2 WHO classification of kidney tumours

Familial renal cancer

Renal cell tumours

Malignant

  Clear cell renal cell carcinoma

  Multilocular clear cell renal cell carcinoma

  Papillary renal cell carcinoma

  Chromophobe renal cell carcinoma

  Carcinoma of the collecting ducts of Bellini

  Renal medullary carcinoma

  Xp11 translocation carcinomas

  Carcinoma associated with neuroblastoma

  Mucinous tubular and spindle cell carcinoma

  Renal cell carcinoma unclassified

Benign

  Papillary adenoma

  Oncocytoma

Metanephric tumours

Metanephric adenoma

Metanephric adenofibroma

Metanephric stromal tumours

Mixed mesenchymal and epithelial tumours

Cystic nephroma

Mixed epithelial and stromal tumour

Synovial sarcoma

Nephroblastic tumours

Nephrogenic rests

Nephroblastoma

Cystic partially differentiated nephroblastoma

Neuroendocrine tumours

Carcinoid

Neuroendocrine carcinoma

Primitive neuroectodermal tumour

Neuroblastoma

Pheochromocytoma

Other tumours

Mesenchymal tumours

Haematopoietic and lymphoid tumours

Germ cell tumours

Metastatic tumours

1.1.2 Malignant renal epithelial tumours

Malignant renal epithelial tumours include the following subtypes:

- Clear cell renal carcinoma (conventional histology)
- Papillary renal cell carcinoma (Type 1 and Type 2)
- Chromophobe renal cell carcinoma
- Collecting duct carcinoma.

1.1.2.1 *Clear cell renal carcinoma*

Clear cell renal carcinoma (CCRC) is the commonest type of renal cancer, accounting for approximately 75% of cases. The classic presentation 'triad' of haematuria, flank pain, and loin mass is notoriously rare, with the majority of cases now being diagnosed incidentally. CCRC is composed of neoplastic cells packed with lipid and glycogen. Histopathological fixation results in the appearance of the 'clear cytoplasm', arranged in either sheets or trabeculae with an abundant fibrovascular stroma, in a pseudoglandular or cystic pattern.

1.1.2.2 *Papillary renal cell carcinoma (Type 1 and Type 2)*

The second most common form of renal cancer is papillary renal cell carcinoma (PRCC), which accounts for 10–15% of cases. Histologically, PRCCs are characterized by lipid-laden macrophages (foamy macrophages) and small calcified concretions (psammoma bodies). They are frequently multifocal and bilateral, and examination of nephrectomy specimens usually identifies multiple papillary renal adenomas that accompany the PRCC. Patients with end-stage kidney disease are at increased risk of developing renal malignancies, particularly of the PRCC type. In contrast to CCRC, PRCCs are often hypovascular and tumour calcification can occur.

There are two distinct subtypes of PRCC with prognostic implications, Type 1 and Type 2. Type 1 PRCC consists of basophilic cells covering thin papillae, is twice as common, and has a better prognosis than Type 2 PRCC which is composed of eosinophilic cells arranged in a pseudostratification architecture.

1.1.2.3 *Chromophobe renal cell carcinoma*

Chromophobe RCC, the third most common carcinoma of the kidney, is a slow growing solid tumour composed of large polygonal tumour cells. On electron microscopy the tumour cells are packed with microvesicles. Chromophobe RCC and oncocytomas are thought to share a common cell of origin, the intercalated cells of the collecting duct, and it is postulated that oncocytomas are the benign counterpart of chromophobe RCC. The prognosis is good.

1.1.2.4 *Collecting duct carcinoma*

Collecting duct carcinoma (also known as Bellini duct carcinomas) and its aggressive variant medullary carcinoma, which is associated with sickle cell trait, are rare accounting for less than 1% of renal tumours.

1.2 **Molecular basis of disease**

- Inherited renal cancer predisposition syndromes
- Mutations in different genes implicated in different histological subtypes of renal cancer
- Defects in –VHL gene underlie hereditary and sporadic CCRC.

Significant insights into the molecular basis of renal cancer tumorigenesis have been made in the past decade. The majority of the advances in our knowledge have been made from studying patients and rare families with inherited risk factors for renal cancer usually occurring as part of a multi-cancer syndrome such as von Hippel–Lindau (VHL) disease (see later). Although only 2% of renal cancers occur in individuals with inherited predisposition, the genetic alterations responsible for the inherited increased risk have also been shown to underlie sporadic cases of renal cancer. Moreover, mutations in several completely distinct genes are implicated in each different histological subtype of renal cancer (Table 1.3).

1.2.1 **Molecular basis of clear cell renal carcinoma**

Mutations in the tumour suppressor VHL gene underlie the inherited multi-cancer VHL disease whereby affected patients can have a very high life-time risk of developing clear cell renal cancer of around 75%.

Table 1.3 Different genetic mutations underlie different histological subtypes of renal cancer		
Histological subtype	**Gene implicated**	**Gene locus**
Clear cell renal carcinoma	von Hippel–Lindau (VHL)	3p25
	Lung cancer tumour suppressor gene region 1 (LCTSGR1)	3p21
	Lung cancer tumour suppressor gene region 2 (LCTSGR2)	3p12
	Fragile histidine triad (FHIT)	3p14
	RAS association domain family 1A (RASSF1A)	3p21
Type 1 papillary renal carcinoma	c-MET	7q31
Type 2 papillary renal carcinoma	Fumarate hydratase (FH)	1q42
Chromophobe renal carcinoma	Birt–Hogg–Dubé (BHD)	17p11
Oncocytoma	BHD	17p11

Other clinical features include haemangioblastomas of the central nervous system (CNS) and retina, pheochromocytomas, pancreatic islet cell tumours, endolymphatic sac tumours, and epididymal cystadenomas. VHL disease can be divided into two main groups depending on the risk of developing pheochromocytoma: families affected by Type 1 VHL disease do not have an increased risk whereas families affected by Type 2 VHL disease are affected by increased susceptibility to pheochromocytomas. Type 2 disease can further be subdivided by families with low risk (Type 2A) or high risk of developing CCRC (Type 2B). Type 2C patients have increased risk of developing pheochromocytomas alone. A third type of VHL disease has recently been recognized (Type 3 disease, also known as Chuvash polycythaemia) whereby affected individuals have erythrocytosis and are characteristically not associated with other classical manifestations of VHL disease. VHL disease affects 1 in 36,000 live births. Type 1 and Type 2 are inherited in an autosomal dominant manner, whereas Type 3 is autosomal recessive, with *de novo* mutations arising in 20% of patients.

The *VHL* gene was cloned in 1993, and resides on the short arm of chromosome 3 (3p25–26). Approximately one-third of patients have *VHL* mutations which are deletions, one-third have missense mutations, and one-third have nonsense or frameshift mutations. Intriguingly, clear genotype–phenotype associations are recognized with Type 1 families tending to have deletions and truncations, Type 2 families generally harbouring missense mutations, and a specific point mutation (598C>T) is identified in Type 3 VHL disease.

The majority of affected individuals inherit a germline mutation in VHL (the first 'hit' in Knudson's classical tumour suppressor two-hit hypothesis) and require somatic inactivation of the remaining wild-type allele (i.e., the second 'hit') for phenotypic manifestations to occur. As is characteristic for inherited cancer susceptibility syndromes, the development of CCRC in VHL patients tends to occur typically a decade or two earlier than those in the sporadic population and are usually multifocal and bilateral. Most important, mutations in the *VHL* gene have been found in approximately 60% of sporadic CCRC, with epigenetic functional silencing by hypermethylation in a further 19% of sporadic cases.

The *VHL* gene encodes two proteins (pVHL30 and pVHL19) that are biologically active and behave similarly, the smaller protein resulting from an alternate translation initiation site. Putative functions of *VHL* include interactions with the β-catenin signalling pathway, fibronectin matrix assembly, atypical protein kinase C, and RNA polymerase II subunits, but the best established function of *VHL* is its central role in cellular oxygen sensing by regulation of the transcription factor hypoxia-inducible factor (HIF). HIF is a heterodimer, consisting of a constitutively expressed β subunit and a regulated α subunit. In normal levels of oxygen tension, specific prolyl residues on the HIF α subunit are hydroxylated and pVHL acts as a recognition component of an E3 ubiquitin ligase complex that binds and targets the prolyl-hydroxylated HIF α subunit for proteosomal degradation. In hypoxia, the hydroxylation of the HIF α subunit is less efficient, resulting in stabilized levels which are able to dimerize with the β subunit forming an active HIF complex to initiate transcription of hypoxic target genes such as *VEGF*, *GLUT1*, and *EPO*. Defective function of pVHL either from mutation or epigenetic silencing will also result in accumulation and stabilization of the α subunit with similar transcriptional consequences. This provides a plausible explanation for the highly vascular nature of VHL defective neoplasms such as CCRC and haemangioblastomas.

It is becoming increasingly clear that other tumour suppressor genes residing on chromosome 3p are important in both VHL defective and competent renal tumourigenesis; these include lung cancer tumour suppressor gene region 1 and 2 (*LCTSGR1* and *LCTSGR2*, 3p21.3 and 3p12, respectively), fragile histidine triad gene (*FHIT*, 3p14), and the RAS association domain family 1A (*RASSF1A*, 3p21).

1.2.2 Molecular basis of PRCC, chromophobe RCC, and oncocytomas

Hereditary PRCC is a rare autosomal dominant hereditary form of Type 1 PRCC with an incidence of approximately 1 in 10 million. Affected individuals inherit activating missense mutations of the *c-MET* proto-oncogene on chromosome 7, and the same genetic alteration has been identified in sporadic cases of Type 1 PRCC. The function of *c-MET* is that of a cell surface receptor for the hepatocyte growth factor/scatter factor (HGF/SF) with diverse downstream effects including increased cell proliferation, motility, and apoptosis.

The hereditary form of Type 2 PRCC is hereditary leiomyomatosis renal cell carcinoma (HLRCC) and is characteristically accompanied by uterine fibroids in affected women and cutaneous leiomyomatosis lesions. Inactivating mutations in the fumarate hydratase (*FH*) gene (chromosome 1q42) underlies HLRCC and is thought to be also important in the sporadic Type 2 PRCC counterpart, although this is not yet clarified.

Birt–Hogg–Dubé syndrome is another rare inherited renal cancer predisposition syndrome associated with hamartomatous tumours of the hair follicle and pulmonary cysts. Affected individuals are at risk of developing bilateral multifocal renal tumours which can be either chromophobe (33%), mixed chromophobe/oncocytic (50%), or more rarely, oncocytoma (7%) or clear cell RCC (5%). Little is known about the *BHD* gene which is located on chromosome 17 and its product, the protein folliculin, and further studies are required to elucidate its functional role in renal tumourigenesis.

References and further reading

Gnarra JR, Tory K, Weng Y, *et al.* (1994). Mutations of the VHL tumour suppressor gene in renal carcinoma. *Nature Genetics*, **7(1)**, 85–90.

Iliopoulos O, Kibel A, Gray S and Kaelin WG Jr (1995). Tumour suppression by the human von Hippel-Lindau gene product. *Nature Medicine*, **1(8)**, 822–6.

Latif F, Tory K, Gnarra J, *et al.* (1993). Identification of the von Hippel-Lindau disease tumor suppressor gene. *Science*, **260(5112)**, 1317–20.

Linehan WM, Walther MM and Zbar B (2003). The genetic basis of cancer of the kidney. *Journal of Urology*, **170(6 Pt 1)**, 2163–72.

Maxwell PH, Wiesener MS, Chang GW, *et al.* (1999). The tumour suppressor protein VHL targets hypoxia-inducible factors for oxygen-dependent proteolysis. *Nature*, **399(6733)**, 271–5.

Mundy AR, Fitzpatrick J, Neal DE and George N (2004). *Scientific basis of urology*, 2nd edn, Chapter 22. Taylor and Francis Ltd: London.

Murai M and Oya M (2004). Renal cell carcinoma: etiology, incidence and epidemiology. *Current Opinion in Urology*, **14(4)**, 229–33.

Renshaw AA (2002). Subclassification of renal cell neoplasms: an update for the practising pathologist. *Histopathology*, **41(4)**, 283–300.

Wang KL, Weinrach DM, Luan C, *et al.* (2007). Renal papillary adenoma—a putative precursor of papillary renal cell carcinoma. *Human Pathology*, **38(2)**, 239–46.

Chapter 2

Radiological assessment

Aslam Sohaib

Key points

- Radiological assessment is central to the multidisciplinary management of a patient with renal cancer
- Imaging is used in the following:
  - Detection and characterization of renal tumour
  - Staging renal cancer
  - Planning surgery
  - Assessment of treatment response
  - Follow up of a patient/detection of recurrent or metastatic disease
- Contrast-enhanced computed tomography (CT) is the main imaging modality used in the evaluation of a patient with renal cancer
- Ultrasound and magnetic resonance imaging are often used as complementary or problem-solving imaging techniques to CT
- Role for positron emission tomography with F-18-2-fluoro-2-deoxyglucose (FDG) is limited as the primary tumour and metastatic disease are often not FDG avid.

2.1 Radiological techniques in the evaluation of renal cancer

2.1.1 Computed tomography

Computed tomography (CT) is the main imaging modality used in the evaluation of a patient with renal cancer. CT images are generated from the attenuation of x-ray beams through the patient. A recent development is the multidetector CT, where a rotation of multiple rows of detector (i.e., 8, 16, 32, or 64) with the x-ray tube around the patient results in multiple slices of images per rotation. Multidetector CT has transformed CT from a purely transaxial cross-sectional imaging to a true three-dimensional (3D) imaging modality that allows viewing of examinations in any plane using multiplanar reformation (MPR). In renal cancer, modern multidetector CT with

MPR imaging allows for better assessment of the disease, especially with respect to surgical planning and staging.

Attention to the imaging technique is essential in evaluating renal masses and the imaging protocol will depend on the clinical question. Scans are performed before the administration of intravenous (IV) contrast to identify calcification and fat within a lesion, and as a baseline to assess enhancement following IV contrast to characterize lesions as solid or cystic. Following IV contrast, images can be obtained as follows:

- Vascular phase images give optimal visualization of aorta and renal arteries and are used for CT arteriography
- Corticomedullary phase images show brisk enhancement of renal cortex and are not often used but may help in the characterization of vascular tumours
- Nephrographic phase. The renal medulla and cortex have a similar degree of enhancement and this phase is best for the detection and characterization renal tumours
- Excretory phase provides urographic images and information relating to the collecting systems and is used for CT urography.

2.1.2 **Ultrasound**

Ultrasound uses high-frequency sound waves to generate images. Ultrasound provides a simple, quick, easy, and cheap method for the assessment of the renal system. Doppler ultrasound techniques use the Doppler effect to show flow by detecting the change in frequency of ultrasound waves in relation to moving structures such as blood. Doppler ultrasound can aid in the assessment of renal lesions and this may be combined with the use of recently developed ultrasound contrast agents. Despite the advances in ultrasound technology, the main role for ultrasound has remained in distinguishing between solid or cystic renal lesions.

2.1.3 **Magnetic resonance imaging**

Magnetic resonance imaging (MRI) uses very strong magnetic field and radiofrequency waves to generate images. The role of MRI is often complementary to CT in the assessment of renal disease. The main advantages of MRI over CT are (i) no use of ionizing radiation and (ii) its greater contrast resolution. Direct multiplanar imaging on MRI used to be an advantage over CT but this is no longer the case with the advent of MPR on multi-detector CT. MRI may be of use in patients unable to receive iodinated IV contrast media due to allergies or renal failure. The advantage of MRI in patients with renal failure is due to the greater contrast resolution of MRI although IV gadolinium is now contraindicated in patients with renal failure. Gadolinium-based contrast media have been implicated in the development of nephrogenic systemic fibrosis (NSF).

Imaging techniques used in MRI are even more important than CT. The complexity and versatility of MRI mean that the imaging protocols are highly dependent on the clinical question. This cannot be overemphasized as the wrong sequences may not address the clinical problem and may require re-imaging. As in CT, it is also possible to obtain angiographic, urographic, and 3D imaging on MRI.

Open magnet systems are available and are used for claustrophobic patients, and usually operate at lower field strengths (<1.0T). Open magnet systems combined with real-time interactive MRI have led to an increasing interest in interventional MRI techniques such as MR-guided biopsies and ablation of tumours.

2.1.4 **Radionuclide imaging**

2.1.4.1 *FDG-PET*

Positron emission tomography (PET) uses radioisotopes that emit positrons for imaging. Much of the initial work on PET was based on PET only scanners which provided planar views of the body with limited anatomical details. However, more recently combined PET–CT scanners allow the PET and CT images to be fused, giving both the functional and anatomical details.

In patients with cancer, F-18-2-fluoro-2-deoxyglucose (FDG) is the most commonly used radiopharmaceutical. FDG is transported into cancer cells like glucose and accumulates within the cell in proportion to the rate of glycolysis. Tumours often exhibit high metabolic rates and show as being FDG avid on PET imaging. However, FDG PET–CT has not yet proven useful in the detection or characterization of renal tumours. The eventual role in recurrent and metastatic renal cancer of FDG PET–CT is yet to be defined.

2.1.4.2 *Other radionuclide imaging*

Bone scintigraphy (with Technetium-99m methylene diphosphonate [99m Tc-MDP]) is used to identify bone metastases in patients with advanced disease. The uptake of the tracer in bone scintigraphy is related to osteoblastic activity and therefore is relatively poor at identifying lytic metastases.

Dimercaptosuccinic acid (DMSA) scans (99mTC-DMSA) are used to quantify viable cortical renal tissues in each kidney and is the most reliable method for measuring split renal function.

2.2 **Detection and characterization of renal tumours**

Renal tumours are often detected incidentally on imaging. The increased use of imaging has resulted in increased detection of smaller and asymptomatic renal tumours.

In suspected renal cell cancer (RCC), the first line of investigation is best performed using CT as staging information is also obtained. Where the lesion remains indeterminate on CT further characterization may be performed using ultrasound or MRI. If after clinical and imaging evaluation of a renal lesion malignancy cannot be excluded, then surgical excision or image-guided biopsy should be performed.

2.2.1 **Solid renal tumours**

If on imaging a lesion is clearly solid, it has traditionally been thought to most likely represent a RCC. More recently, however, there has been increasing evidence that not all solid lesions are RCCs (especially smaller tumours).

The only solid renal masses that can be reliably differentiated from renal cancer on CT or MRI are angiomyolipomas (AMLs). Macroscopic fat present in most AMLs has a characteristic appearance on CT and MRI. Occasionally, AML may contain such small amounts of fat that the fatty area cannot be identified on imaging. These are known as 'renal AML with minimal fat' and cannot be distinguished from malignant renal tumours.

The other common benign solid renal tumour is an oncocytoma. Imaging may reveal a central stellate scar in oncocytomas but this is not always a reliable sign and it is not possible to distinguish between an oncocytoma and a renal cancer on imaging alone.

Several studies have tried to distinguish between the different histological subtypes of renal cancer using imaging. For example, clear cell RCC often enhances more quickly and intensely than other tumours. However, none of the imaging features are reliable enough to avoid biopsy or surgery.

2.2.2 **Cystic renal tumours**

Cystic renal lesions are classified using the Bosniak system according to CT features (Table 2.1). The Bosniak classification represents an imaging and clinical management system and is not a pathological classification. Increasing complexity of the cyst is associated with increase in the risk of malignancy. Category I and II cysts are always benign and do not require further imaging follow up. Category IIF requires imaging follow up as a few may be malignant (~5%). Category III and IV are generally treated surgically as about half of all category III lesions are malignant and all category IV lesions are cystic cancers.

Table 2.1 The Bosniak cyst classification	
Category	**CT findings**
Category I	**Benign simple cysts:** Hairline thin walls. No septa, calcifications, solid components. No enhancement.
Category II	**Benign cystic lesions:** Thin walls. Hairline thin septa. Fine calcification in wall/septa. Minimal enhancement. Hyperdense non-enhancing cysts also included (<3cm).
Category IIF	**Complicated cystic lesions:** Multiple hairline thin septa; there may be minimal thickening of wall or septa, which may contain calcification that may be thick and nodular; there are no enhancing soft tissue components. Hyperdense non-enhancing cyst >3cm
Category III	**Indeterminate masses:** Thick irregular walls or septa that show enhancement.
Category IV	**Malignant cystic masses:** Thick irregular walls or septa that show enhancement, with enhancing soft tissue components.

2.2.3 FDG-PET in characterizing renal tumours

FDG-PET does not yet have a proven role in the detection or characterization of renal tumours. RCC may show a low-grade uptake of FDG that makes it difficult to differentiate from normal renal parenchyma. Furthermore, urinary excretion of FDG limits the evaluation of renal masses PET images. The sensitivity of FDG-PET for the detection of renal cancer is in the region of 60–70%. FDG-PET can show false positive results in AML and oncocytoma. Overall FDG-PET has no advantage over contrast-enhanced CT for primary lesion characterization.

2.3 Staging

2.3.1 Staging system

The current version of the 2002 TNM staging of the American Joint Committee on Cancer (AJCC) and the International Union Against Cancer (UICC) is shown in Tables 2.2 and 2.3. The Robson classification is an alternative staging system no longer used but still referred to in many texts (Table 2.4).

Table 2.2 TNM staging classification

Primary tumour	
TX	Primary tumour cannot be assessed
T0	No evidence of primary tumour
T1	Tumour ≤7cm in greatest diameter, limited to the kidney
T1a	Tumour ≤4cm in greatest diameter, limited to the kidney
T1b	Tumour >4cm but ≤7cm in greatest diameter, limited to the kidney
T2	Tumour >7cm in greatest diameter, limited to the kidney
T3	Tumour extends into the major veins or invades adrenal gland or perinephric tissues but not beyond Gerota's fascia
T3a	Tumour invades adrenal gland or perinephric tissues but not beyond Gerota's fascia
T3b	Tumour extends into the renal veins or vena cava below the diaphragm
T3c	Tumour extends into vena cava above the diaphragm or invades wall of the vena cava
T4	Tumour invades beyond Gerota's fascia
Regional lymph nodes	
NX	Regional nodes cannot be assessed
N0	No regional lymph node metastasis
N1	Metastasis to a single regional node
N2	Metastasis to more than one regional node
Regional lymph nodes	
MX	Distant metastasis cannot be assessed
M0	No distant metastasis
M1	Distant metastasis

Table 2.3 TNM stage groupings

Stage			
I	T1	N0	M0
II	T2	N0	M0
III	T1 or T2	N1	M0
	T3	N0 or N1	M0
IV	T4	N0 or N1	M0
	Any T	N2	M0
	Any T	Any N	M1

Table 2.4 Robson classification versus TNM system

Robson grade	Disease extent	TNM
I	Tumour confined to the kidney	T1-T2
II	Tumour spread to perinephric tissues but not beyond Gerota's fascia	T3a
IIIA	Tumour spread to renal vein or vena cava	T3b
IIIB	Tumour spread to local nodes	N1-2
IIIC	Tumour spread to local vessels and nodes	T3b, N1-2
IVA	Tumour spread to adjacent organs	T4
IVB	Distant metastases	M1

Staging in renal cancer is usually performed using CT, as this allows the assessment of the primary tumour, nodal and metastatic disease, as well as an evaluation of the contralateral kidney. Coronal and sagittal reformats are helpful in assessing tumour and the vascular anatomy. MRI may be used as an alternative to CT for staging but its main use is in the assessment of the extent of tumour thrombus in the inferior vena cava (IVC) and evaluating any equivocal lesion on the staging CT. Ultrasound has only a very limited role in tumour staging, as abdominal bowel gas will often limit the evaluation. FDG-PET is not routinely used in staging renal cancer.

2.3.2 Primary tumour

CT is excellent at assessing tumours confined to the renal capsule. Staging perinephric invasion (T3a disease) is a common source of staging error. An enhancing perinephric mass is a highly specific finding, but many patients with perinephric invasion may not have this feature on CT or MRI. Other less specific findings of capsular invasion include an indistinct tumour margin, and thickening or stranding of the perinephric tissues.

Venous extension of tumour (stage T3b-c disease) can be assessed on ultrasound, CT, or MRI. Sonography is highly accurate at assessing tumour thrombus within the IVC if the examination is technically adequate. Transoesophageal or transthoracic sonography may be helpful if tumour thrombus is suspected to extend into the right atrium. Colour Doppler assessment improves overall accuracy in assessing tumour extent. On contrast-enhanced CT, the presence of a persistent filling defect within the renal vein or IVC is a sensitive and specific sign of thrombus. Sagittal and coronal reformatted images allow determination of the upper extent of thrombus. MRI is probably the best technique in delineating the extent of IVC thrombus. Furthermore, tumoural invasion of the IVC wall can sometimes be predicted using MRI. Tumour extending through the wall allows a definitive diagnosis, but altered wall thickness and vessel wall enhancement may also be features.

2.3.3 **Lymph nodes**

Spread of renal cancer to regional nodes includes renal hilar, paraaortic and paracaval nodes. There is an increase in the incidence of reactive nodes in the presence of necrotic tumour or venous thrombus. Lymphadenopathy in the chest represents distant metastasis.

The presence of lymph nodes disease is a poor prognostic factor. On both CT and MRI, the diagnosis of lymph node involvement is based on size criteria, which has well-known limitations. CT and MRI are unable to identify metastases in normal-sized lymph nodes, and both are unable to distinguish enlarged nodes due to reactive change from enlargement due to malignant infiltration. However, metastatic tumour is invariably present in nodes larger than 2cm. Overall accuracy of CT staging of lymph nodes has been reported as approximately 70–80%, and MRI is at least comparable to that of CT.

2.3.4 **Metastases**

The assessment of metastatic disease is usually performed using contrast-enhanced CT of the body with MRI of the brain and a radionuclide bone scintigraphy performed as clinically indicated. Distant metastases occur most commonly due to haematogenous spread and are often multifocal. They occur most frequently in the lungs with other favoured sites including bone, liver, contralateral kidney, adrenals, and brain.

Pulmonary metastases are usually multiple soft tissue density lesions classically described as 'cannon ball' metastases on a chest radiograph, but are more frequently smaller and of varying size. The advent of multidetector CT is likely to increase the detection of small pulmonary metastases. Other patterns of disease in the chest include mediastinal adenopathy, pleural disease including effusions and lymphangitis carcinomatosa, and rarely endobronchial metastases.

Bone metastases are typically lytic and expansile and occur mainly in the axial skeleton, though may affect the diaphyses of the long bones. Plain radiography and bone scintigraphy are usually used to identify bone metastases in patients with advanced disease. However, bone scintigraphy is poor at identifying lytic metastases and in this regard whole-body MRI is more sensitive than bone scintigraphy.

Liver metastases are typically hypodense on CT, but renal cancer is one of the few malignancies that can produce hypervascular liver metastases. MRI is useful in evaluating the liver when a lesion is equivocal on CT or ultrasound.

Metastatic disease to the brain and central nervous system is best assessed using MRI.

The role of FDG-PET in the assessment for metastases in renal cancer is unclear but is sometimes used when the findings on CT are equivocal. FDG-PET has limited sensitivity for small metastases, and a negative FDG-PET does not exclude a malignancy but a positive FDG-PET should be considered suspicious.

2.4 **Surgical planning**

A number of imaging findings are vital in the preoperative evaluation and include the position of the kidney, the tumour size and precise location with respect to the renal surface, collecting system, and the vessels. For example, the most suitable lesion for nephron-sparing surgery is small (<4cm), polar, cortical, and distant from the renal hilum and collecting system. This information can be obtained using CT or MRI. Coronal and sagittal reformats are essential in assessing the tumour and the vascular anatomy if nephron-sparing surgery is planned for the demonstration of vascular anomalies. The decision to perform partial versus total nephrectomy may also be influenced by renal function, and differential renal function can be assessed using DMSA scan.

2.5 **Response assessment**

The advent of new drug treatments in metastatic renal cancer has meant that response assessment to therapy is now more frequently needed. As there are no other tumour makers in renal cancer, imaging is central to the response evaluation.

2.5.1 **RECIST**

The standard endpoint to assess treatment response is to measure the change in tumour size using the RECIST (Response Evaluation Criteria in Solid Tumours) criteria (see Table 2.5). RECIST criteria have recently been updated to version 1.1. The National Cancer Institute (NCI), and the European Organization for Research and Treatment of Cancer (EORTC) have adopted RECIST criteria for response evaluation.

2.6 **Follow up/surveillance**

There is no firm consensus on the follow up and surveillance of patients treated for renal cancer; however, imaging does play an important role in most follow-up protocols. Again the frequency, duration, and imaging modality used varies. Most of the strategies are based on the likelihood of developing relapse or metastases (e.g., nomogram such as Mayo scoring system may be used to assess the risk of metastases following nephrectomy). Where the likelihood of relapse is low, use of imaging is minimal with chest x-ray used to look for pulmonary metastases and other imaging based on symptoms. Where the risk is intermediate or high, CT of chest and abdomen is the investigation of choice.

Table 2.5 **RECIST 1.1 criteria**	
Response categories	
Complete response (CR)	Complete resolutions of all target lesions
Partial response (PR)	At least 30% reduction in tumour size
Stable disease	Neither PR nor PD

*Non-measurable lesions are as follows: small lesions, bone lesions, meningeal lesions, ascites, pleural or pericardial effusion, lymphangitis, and cystic or necrotic lesions.

References and further reading

Eisenhauer EA, Therasse P, Bogaerts J, *et al.* (2009). New response evaluation criteria in solid tumors: revised RECIST guideline (version 1.1). *Eur J Cancer*, **45(2)**, 228–47.

Griffin N, Gore ME and Sohaib SA (2007). Imaging in metastatic renal cell carcinoma. *American Journal of Roentgenology*, **189(2)**, 360–70.

Israel GM and Bosniak MA (2005). How I do it: evaluating renal masses. *Radiology*, **236(2)**, 441–50.

Patel U, ed. (2007). *Carcinoma of the kidney. Series: contemporary issues in cancer imaging*. Cambridge University Press, Cambridge.

Reznek RH and Webb JAW (2004). Renal tumours. In JE Husband, RH Reznek, eds. *Imaging in oncology*, pp. 273–305. Taylor and Francis, Abingdon.

Sobin LH and Wittekind C (2002). *International Union Against Cancer (UICC) TNM classification of malignant tumours*, 6th edn. Wiley-Liss, New York.

Chapter 3

Assessment of treatment options in renal cancer

Martin Gore and Sheeba Irshad

> **Key points**
>
> - Several models have been developed as prognostic tools to select patients for treatment strategies, analyse results of clinical trials, and give information to patients regarding prognosis
> - For localized and locally advanced tumours, surgery is the gold standard
> - Observation remains standard of care after nephrectomy but results of current adjuvant phase III trials are awaited
> - Published phase III trials have established the novel targeted agents as standard of care for patients with metastatic renal cell carcinoma (mRCC)
> - Only selected patients with mRCC, revealing a good-risk profile, and clear cell subtype histology have any chance of deriving clinical benefit from immunotherapy.

There have been a number of advances in the management of renal cell carcinoma (RCC) over the past 20 years. These include advances in surgical options, immunotherapy, and targeted therapies.

3.1 Prognostic factors and patient selection

The use of integrated prognostic systems or nomograms provide an important tool to select patients for treatment strategies, analyse results of clinical trials, and give information to patients regarding prognosis. Since 2001, several models have been developed as prognostic tools, containing many available clinical and pathological findings.

Factors influencing prognosis can be classified broadly into the following categories:

- Anatomical:
  - TNM staging system—includes tumour size, venous invasion, renal capsule invasion, adrenal involvement, lymph node, and distant metastases
  - The presence of lymph node metastases is a reliable predictor of a poor outcome in locally advanced RCC.
- Histological:
  - Two main subtypes of RCC have been established: clear cell (80% of RCCs) and non-clear cell (papillary Type 1 and 2, chromophobe, collecting duct, and unclassified carcinomas)
  - A number of studies have suggested the use of histological diagnosis as a predictor of responsiveness to immunotherapy
    —Clear cell histology is associated with better responses to treatment with interleukin-2 (IL-2) immunotherapy compared to non-clear cell histology
    —Patients with tumours that have papillary, >50% granular or no alveolar features, respond poorly to IL-2
  - Type 1 papillary RCC are low-grade tumours with a chromophilic cytoplasm and a favourable prognosis, and Type 2 are generally high-grade tumours with eosinophilic cytoplasm and are associated with a higher risk of metastatic progression and poor prognosis.
- Molecular:
  - Increased understanding of molecular signalling pathways involved in the pathogenesis of RCC has prompted a more thorough analysis of the proteins expressed on the tumour cells
  - Carbonic anhydrase IX (CA IX):
    —A transmembrane protein that is thought to play a role in the regulation of cell proliferation under hypoxic conditions
    —Present in 94% of clear cell RCCs, reduced CA IX levels have been associated with poor prognosis in patients with metastatic disease
    —Tissue specimens from patients with good pathological prognosis alone or intermediate pathological prognosis with high CA IX expression levels correlated with 96% of responders to IL-2 treatment. Thus, CA IX has emerged as a strong candidate for predicting response, progression, and survival in patients with metastatic RCC (mRCC) treated with IL-2
  - Some of the other molecular markers currently under investigation are CA XII, VEGF family, IGF-1, and Ki-67.

- Clinical:
  —Many clinical features have been identified that may influence survival in patient. Performance status and the number of metastatic sites may be the most relevant
  —Analysis of outcome by prognostic factors is complicated by the lack of a common system for prospectively identifying and stratifying patients and analysing the findings
  —Moreover, differences in the findings of studies conducted to date (nearly all of which have been retrospective) suggest that large, prospective studies are required to usefully define prognostic clinical features.

3.1.1 Current prognostic models

Several groups have sought to combine several prognostic factors to provide superior predictive information for individual patients.

3.1.1.1 UCLA Integrated Staging System

The UCLA Integrated Staging System (UISS) is the main validated system when all renal cancer subtypes are grouped together. UISS uses stage (1997 TNM), Fuhrman's grade, and the Eastern Cooperative Oncology Group (ECOG) performance status to stratify patients into groups at low, intermediate, and high risk (Table 3.1). Notably, the UISS system is being used to select patients in two phase III adjuvant trials: S-TRAC and ASSURE (see Section 3.3).

3.1.1.2 The Leibovich risk model

Developed at the Mayo Clinic, this model aims to predict progression in patients with clinically localized, clear cell RCC who undergo radical nephrectomy. It integrates the prognostic features of pathological stage, primary tumour size, nuclear grade, and tumour necrosis into a single score: the SSIGN (stage, size, grade, and necrosis) score.

The SSIGN score has recently been shown to have a higher prognostic accuracy than UISS in the series of surgically treated clear cell RCC, suggesting a larger use of the SSIGN score in the design of randomized clinical trials with the novel targeted therapies.

The SSIGN score is being used to select patients for the SORCE trial (Section 3.3).

3.1.1.3 The Memorial Sloan-Kettering Cancer Center (MSKCC) prognostic model

Developed from a retrospective study by Motzer and colleagues, this prognostic model is commonly used to stratify patients entering clinical trials of first-line treatment. Under this model, patients are categorized into favourable, intermediate, or poor prognostic group based on five risk factors as follows:

- Karnofsky performance status (<80%)

Table 3.1 The UCLA integrated staging system (UISS)					
Patient group		**Prognostic group**			
		T stage	Fuhrman's grade	ECOG status	5-year disease specific survival
Localized disease (N_0, M_0)	Low risk	1	1–2	0	91.1%
	Intermediate risk	1	1–2	1 or more	80.4%
		1	3–4	Any	
		2	Any	Any	
		3	1	Any	
		3	2–4	Any	
	High	3	2–4	1 or more	54.7%
		4	Any	Any	
Metastatic disease	Low risk	N_1M_0	Any	Any	32%
		N_2M_0/M_1	1–2	0	
	Intermediate risk	N_2M_0/M_1	1–2	1 or more	19.5%
			3	0, 1 or more	
			4	0	
	High	N_2M_0/M_1	4	1 or more	0%

22

- Elevated lactate dehydrogenase (>1.5 times the upper limit of normal)
- Low haemoglobin (< normal)
- High 'corrected' calcium
- Absence of prior nephrectomy/initiation of interferon-α (IFN-α) within less than 1 year of diagnosis (modified MSKCC).

Patients with no risk factors (favourable-risk) had a median survival of 20 months, one to two risk factors (intermediate-risk) 10 months, and 4 months for those with three or more risk factors (poor-risk). Furthermore, a large prospective study conducted by the Groupe Français d'Immunothérapie identified predictive factors of rapid progression under treatment. Adverse features include the following:

- Presence of hepatic metastases
- Elevated neutrophil count
- Less than 12 months from diagnosis of the primary tumour to the development of metastatic disease
- Two or more metastatic sites.

Patients with at least three of these adverse prognostic factors have a greater than 80% probability of rapid progression despite cytokine treatment.

The addition of three other independent immunological parameters (blood neutrophil count, presence of intratumoural neutrophils, and intratumoural CD57+ natural killer cell count) to prognostic models based on clinical risk factors have been shown to identify subgroups of patients amongst those with favourable clinical features. Estimated 5-year survival rates for the subgroups based on this combined immunological–clinical model were 60%, 25%, and 0% for patients with zero, one, and two to three immunological risk factors, respectively. Investigations into new prognostic models based on clinical factors supplemented with immunological factors are strongly encouraged for those undergoing immunotherapy.

Most prognostic models have focused largely on patient selection for immunotherapy (summarized in Table 3.2); however, in this new era of targeted therapies this field is rapidly evolving, and new prognostic or predictive models for patients treated with these compounds is an important research imperative. Such a model has been proposed, based on the outcome data from the pivotal phase III sunitinib versus IFN trial, using a nomogram for predicting the probability of 12-month progression-free survival (PFS) for patients who received sunitinib therapy. It takes into account a number of parameters (corrected serum calcium, the number of metastatic sites, haemoglobin levels, prior nephrectomy, the presence of lung and liver metastases, thrombocytosis, performance status, time from diagnosis to treatment, and serum levels of alkaline phosphatase and lactate dehydrogenase).

23

Table 3.2 Cytokine therapy for metastatic RCC	
Patients likely to benefit	**Patients unlikely to benefit**
• 'Good' prognosis	• 'Intermediate' or 'poor' prognosis
• Nephrectomy	

• Positive histology
  • clear cell with alveolar features
  • lack of granular or papillary features
	• Negative histology
	  • non-clear cell
	  • granular or papillary features

• Immunological markers
  • low neutrophil count
  • lack of intratumoural neutrophils
  • high intratumoural CD57+ T-cells
  • low regulatory T-cell count after treatment
	• Immunological markers
	  • high neutrophil count
	  • presence of intratumoural neutrophils
	  • low intratumoural CD57+ T-cells
	  • high regulatory T-cell count after treatment

• Pathological markers
  • high CA IX expression
	• Pathological markers
	  • low CA IX expression

3.2 Surgical options for RCC

There is an increasing incidence of localized tumours which are often found incidentally on imaging as small, enhancing renal masses. Current options for the management of these small tumours vary between watchful waiting and surgical treatment. At present, surgery remains the gold standard for localized or locally advanced tumours. There are, however, now several surgical options.

3.2.1 Radical nephrectomy

Open radical nephrectomy is reserved for large (>7cm) tumours, and tumours invading the renal vein or inferior vena cava. If successfully removed, the likelihood of recurrence in the renal bed has been reported to be 2–3%.

Laparoscopic nephrectomy is becoming increasingly established as a better option than open nephrectomy. Relative contraindications are large venous thrombus, adjacent organ involvement, and widespread metastatic disease.

Lymph node dissection is not considered therapeutic but does provide prognostic information because virtually all patients with nodal involvement subsequently relapse with distant metastases despite lymphadenectomy.

Other indications for radical nephrectomy include the following:

- Patients with metastatic disease as a palliative procedure in cases of intractable pain and bleeding
- Randomized phase III studies by the Southwest Oncology Group (SWOG 8949) and the European Organization for the Research and Treatment of Cancer have demonstrated a survival benefit for patients with mRCC that undergo cytoreductive nephrectomy before the administration of systemic immunotherapy with IFN. It is felt that surgery should be offered for all eligible patients with a good performance status
- Disadvantages of cytoreductive nephrectomy for metastatic disease include the following:
  - Inevitable surgical morbidity and complications. Mortality is small but may be difficult to eliminate completely because many patients with advanced mRCC are in poor condition
  - Delay in systemic therapy. Earlier non-randomized studies on cytoreductive nephrectomy have shown that almost one-third of the patients have been unable to receive postoperative immunotherapy.

3.2.2 Partial nephrectomy

Partial nephrectomy is a nephron-sparing procedure for patients with small localized tumours, although debate remains regarding the 'cut-off' level for tumour size. In patients with a solitary tumour of less than 4cm maximum diameter, nephron-sparing surgery provides recurrence-free and long-term survival rates similar to those observed after a radical surgical procedure. Lesions larger than 4cm (up to 7cm in greatest dimensions), especially at the poles of the kidney, are sometimes offered a partial nephrectomy with an intensified follow up due to an increased risk of intrarenal recurrences.

Other indications for partial nephrectomy include the following:

• Patients who would otherwise be rendered anephric postoperatively thus necessitating dialysis. These include RCC in a solitary kidney, bilateral lesions or significant preoperative renal insufficiency.

3.2.3 Minimally invasive ablative techniques

Minimally invasive ablative techniques are still regarded as experimental treatment options for kidney cancer and are mainly indicated in patients with a poor performance status with smaller peripheral tumours, or those with multiple tumours in the kidney. Tissue is destroyed *in situ* by techniques such as cryotherapy, radiofrequency, or microwave ablation. Potential advantages include reduced morbidity, outpatient therapy, and the ability to treat high-risk surgical patients.

3.2.4 Metastasectomy

Accumulated evidence from many studies, although retrospective in character, advocates aggressive surgery for metastases because it has been shown to increase survival, especially in patients with solitary metastasis. Many studies report 5-year survival rates in the range of 35% after such surgery.

The European guidelines state that there is a role for metastasectomy in patients with RCC in order to improve the clinical prognosis.

3.2.4.1 Lung metastases

In case of solitary lung metastases, 5-year survival rates after first and even consequent complete resections have been reported as high as >40%. Favourable prognostic features in addition to complete resection include solitary metastasis, absence of metastatic regional and mediastinal lymph nodes, and a long disease-free interval from nephrectomy for primary tumour to appearance of pulmonary metastases. In selected patients a 5-year survival rate of >50% is reached.

Adjuvant treatment with IFN has been shown in studies to increase morbidity and is not routinely recommended after resection of pulmonary metastases. Rather, such patients should be involved in clinical trials testing newer agents.

3.2.4.2 Bone metastases

A recent study from the M.D. Anderson Cancer Center reported that patients with solitary metastasis treated by various orthopaedic procedures had a significantly better survival rate than patients with multiple metastasis (78% at 1-year and 35% at 5-year survival).

Supported by other smaller studies, it is advocated that solitary bone metastases should be treated surgically whenever technically feasible due to the eventual possibility of prolonging survival as well as quality-of-life aspects such as stabilization of an extremity and alleviation of pain.

3.2.4.3 Brain metastases

Patients with untreated brain metastases seldom survive longer than a few months.

Whole-brain radiation is of limited efficacy. Better alternatives are surgical excision or radiosurgery by using a gamma knife.

Studies focused on operatively treated RCC brain metastases have reported overall median survival from the diagnosis of brain metastasis as high as 12 months. No difference is seen between patients with solitary or multiple brain metastases.

Postoperative radiation has not been shown to have any effect on the outcome.

Gamma knife surgery can lead to good local control and can have a favourable impact on survival despite the fact that complete disappearance of brain metastases by this method is relatively rare.

3.3 Medical options for treatment of RCC

3.3.1 Adjuvant setting

Twenty to thirty per cent of patients with localized tumours experience relapse after surgical excision. The median time to relapse after surgery is 1–2 years.

Currently, outside of controlled clinical trials, there are no indications for adjuvant therapy in patients who have undergone a complete resection of their tumour.

Randomized trials comparing adjuvant IFN-α or high-dose IL-2 with observation alone in patients who had locally advanced, completely resected RCC have not yet demonstrated clear evidence of clinical benefit.

Molecular targeted therapies may offer a new approach for adjuvant therapy of this disease. The clinical benefit and tolerability of these agents as adjuvant therapies are being investigated in three ongoing phase III trials, all with the primary end point of disease-free survival (DFS):

- **S-TRAC**—a randomized double-blind phase III study of 1-year adjuvant sunitinib versus placebo in subjects with high-risk RCC as defined by the UISS
- **ASSURE (ECOG 2805)**—double-blind, multicentre study to assess the effect of adjuvant sunitinib versus adjuvant sorafenib versus

placeholder in patients with non-mRCC. It is designed to include potentially curable patients at the highest risk for recurrence based on existing postoperative nomograms

- **SORCE (MRC trial)**—a three-arm study comparing 3 years of sorafenib therapy, 1 year of sorafenib therapy plus 2 years of placebo therapy, and 3 years of placebo therapy in patients with resected primary RCC at high or intermediate risk of relapse according to the Leibovich model.

3.3.2 **Metastatic setting**

Systemic treatment options for mRCC have been limited until recently to cytokine therapy and clinical trials of novel agents. This has changed in the past 1–2 years.

3.3.2.1 Immunotherapy

Spontaneous remissions reported in some patients with mRCC have been thought to be immune-mediated and have provided the basis for immunotherapeutic approaches.

Until recently immunotherapy, principally with IFN-α or high-dose IL-2, has been considered as the standard first-line treatment for patients with mRCC.

As discussed in Section 3.1, it appears however that only a relatively small proportion of highly selected 'good prognosis' group of patients with metastatic clear cell renal carcinoma benefit from cytokine therapy (see Table 3.2):

- The recent PERCY Quattro study demonstrated that patients with intermediate prognosis (>1 metastatic site and Karnofsky score ≥ 80) did not have any survival benefit for cytokine therapy
- A study conducted by the Groupe Français d'Immunothérapie also reported that patients with a poor prognosis (>1 metastatic site, liver involvement, and <1 year from primary tumour to appearance of metastatic disease) had very little chance of benefiting from cytokine therapy.

Although about 8% of patients treated with high-dose IL-2 in the randomized controlled trials have a durable complete remission, the high incidence of toxicity associated with its administration is not trivial. It can only be delivered in specialist centres with facilities for appropriate supportive care, highlighting the importance of patient selection for this treatment.

It should be noted, however, that even in individuals with a favourable group for cytokine therapy, it may be contraindicated in certain patients (Table 3.3).

Table 3.3 Contraindications to cytokine therapy

	IFN-α	IL-2
Contraindications	Autoimmune hepatitis Hepatic decompensation (Child-Pugh class A and B)	Abnormal thallium stress test Abnormal pulmonary function tests Organ allografts Prior drug-related toxicities/sensitivities
Precautions	Neuropsychiatric disorders Autoimmune disorders Ischaemic disorders Infectious disorders	Autoimmune disorders Ischaemic disorders Infectious disorders

The responses seen in patients to immunomodulatory cytokines have provided the rationale for other immunologic strategies for patients with RCC. These potential therapies include the following:

- Allogeneic hematopoietic stem cell transplantation (HSCT)
- Tumour vaccines:
  - Cell-based—for example, dendritic cell, autologous tumour cell
  - Non-cell-based—for example, heat shock proteins, cytotoxic T lymphocyte (CTL) epitope peptide vaccines.

3.3.2.2 Chemotherapy

Renal cell carcinoma is considered resistant to standard cytotoxic or DNA-targeted therapy, with response rates of 4–18% for single agent or combination therapy. The reason for this is thought to be that RCCs develop from the proximal tubules, and these have high levels of expression of the multiple-drug resistance protein P-glycoprotein (gp-170). This protein is thought to have an important role in the mechanisms involved in chemoresistance.

Vinblastine, 5-fluorouracil (5-FU), and fluoropyrimidines are the most effective single agents for mRCC. Combinations of various chemotherapeutic agents have not been shown to improve efficacy compared to monotherapy. Combination therapy with cytokines have been shown to moderately improve the response rate and in some studies, PFS. Chemotherapy is generally used in combination with other therapies or reserved for patients entering clinical trials.

3.3.2.3 Targeted therapies

Recent advances in understanding the molecular biology of kidney cancer have resulted in the development of new drugs that target aberrant molecular pathways associated with this malignancy, resulting in a dramatic change in the management of mRCC.

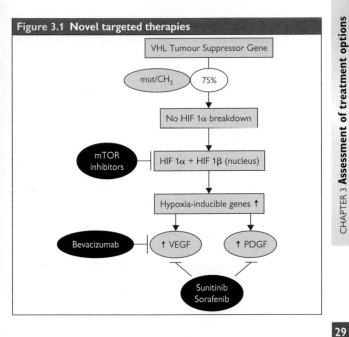

Figure 3.1 Novel targeted therapies

Inactivating mutations of the von Hippel–Lindau (*VHL*) tumour suppressor gene have been found in over 75% of sporadic clear cell RCCs, resulting in increased transcription of hypoxia-inducible genes encoding vascular endothelial growth factor (VEGF), platelet-derived growth factor (PDGF), and transforming growth factor-α (TGFα). Tyrosine kinases are essential enzymes for these growth factors to catalyse the phosphorylation of signalling molecules and in tumours, this results in increased cellular proliferation, survival, and angiogenesis. Hence, inhibitors of tyrosine kinase activity have provided attractive therapeutic targets for combating RCC (Figure 3.1).

To date, four such agents have been approved by the Food and Drug Administration (FDA) following publication of several critical phase III trials for the treatment of advanced RCC: sunitinib malate, sorafenib tosylate, temsirolimus, and bevacizumab with IFN-α (see Table 3.4). These clinical studies have yielded such convincing results that, in addition to their recent approval for use in mRCC, these agents have been incorporated into recently revised EAU guidelines on RCC and the United States National Comprehensive Cancer Network (NCCN) guidelines. There is, however, still a need for additional prospective trials to clarify whether patients with metastatic non-clear cell RCC may also benefit from targeted agents.

Table 3.4 Summary of Level 1 evidence for the management of mRCC			
Treatment line	Prognostic Group		
	Good	Intermediate	Poor
First line	Sunitinib	Sunitinib	Temsirolimus
	Bevacizumab and IFN-α	Bevacizumab and IFN-α	
	Pazopanib	Pazopanib	
	IFN-α or HD IL-2*		
Second line			
Prior cytokine therapy	Sorafenib	Sorafenib	No evidence
	Pazopanib	Pazopanib	
Prior TKI therapy	Everolimus	Everolimus	No evidence

3.3.3 First-line setting

3.3.3.1 Sunitinib

Sunitinib is an orally bioavailable, small multitargeted kinase inhibitor which selectively inhibits PDGF receptor, VEGF receptor, foetal liver tyrosine kinase-3 (Flt-3), and stem cell growth factor c-KIT, resulting in the inhibition of angiogenesis and cell proliferation.

A recent large multicentre, randomized phase III trial established sunitinib as the standard of care for first-line treatment for good- and intermediate-risk patients with mRCC. It demonstrated a significant improvement in PFS, objective response rates, and an overall survival for sunitinib-treated patients in comparison with IFN-α in treatment-naive patients with clear cell mRCC. This study was critical in the approval of sunitinib by NICE in February 2009.

Sunitinib has an acceptable safety profile, with the majority of toxicities reported as mild to moderate. However, the main precautions to consider before starting a patient on sunitinib are summarized in Table 3.5.

- **Hypertension**—Trials have reported an incidence of hypertension in sunitinib-treated patients compared with patients on IFN-α. In cases of severe hypertension (>200mmHg systolic or 110mmHg diastolic), temporary suspension of sunitinib is recommended until hypertension is controlled

- **QT interval prolongation**—Torsades de pointes has been observed in <0.1% of sunitinib-exposed patients. Special consideration should be paid to patients with a known history of QT interval prolongation, or those taking antiarrhythmics, or patients with relevant pre-existing cardiac disease, bradycardia, or electrolyte disturbances

Table 3.5 Safety profile for sunitinib

Precautions with sunitinib

Contraindications
- Paediatric use: the safety and efficacy have not been established
- Hypersensitivity to sunitinib
- Cardiac events, pulmonary embolism, or cerebrovascular events within the previous 12 months
- Severe uncontrolled hypertension (>200mmHg systolic or 110mmHg diastolic)
- Nephrotic syndrome.

Cautions
- History of QT interval prolongation, or those taking antiarrhythmics, or patients with relevant pre-existing cardiac disease, bradycardia, or electro-lyte disturbances
- Concomitant treatment with potent CYP3A4 inhibitors, which may increase sunitinib plasma concentrations
- Proteinuria—monitor for worsening proteinuria while on treatment.

- **Cardiovascular disease**—A decline in left ventricular ejection fraction has been observed in some patients. In the presence of clinical manifestations of congestive heart failure, discontinuation is recommended. Patients with a history of cardiac events, pulmonary embolism, or cerebrovascular events within the previous 12 months should probably be excluded from the therapy.

3.3.3.2 Bevacizumab

Bevacizumab is a recombinant monoclonal antibody that binds VEGF, thus blocking its interaction with the VEGF receptor.

Two phase III trials (the Roche-sponsored AVOREN trial, and Cancer and Leukaemia Group B 90206) randomized previously un-treated patients with mRCC to IFN-α treatment, with or without bevacizumab. In the AVOREN study, combination therapy was superior to IFN-α alone, both in terms of overall response rate and median PFS. No new side effects were observed with the combination compared to that anticipated with each agent alone. However, questions remain about whether bevacizumab was the major source of activity in this combination, as neither trial had a bevacizumab alone arm.

Therefore, the combination of bevacizumab and IFN-α can be considered as a possible alternative to sunitinib as a first-line therapy for patients with mRCC.

Contraindications and cautions to consider before starting a patient on bevacizumab are summarized in Table 3.6.

Table 3.6 Precautions with bevacizumab
Contraindications
• Hypersensitivity to bevacizumab
• Untreated central nervous system (CNS) metastases
• Haemoptysis
• Less than 28 days following major surgery—risk of gastrointestinal perforation and wound dehiscence
• Pregnancy—tetratogenic.
Cautions
• History of arterial thromboembolism or significant cardiovascular disease
• Coagulopathies (congenital, acquired, or therapeutic)
• Hypertension.

3.3.3.3 Temsirolimus

Temsirolimus is an inhibitor of mammalian target of rapamycin (mTOR), which is a non-receptor tyrosine kinase. Activation of mTOR results in multiple tumour-promoting intracellular signalling pathways, including elevated levels of HIF-1α gene expression, de-regulation of cell growth, and angiogenic mechanisms.

A randomized phase III trial comparing temsirolimus as a single agent versus temsirolimus plus IFN-α versus IFN-α alone in previously untreated with poor-risk features, as defined by MSKCC criteria, reported a significant improvement in OS in the temsirolimus alone arm. The combination treatment did not result in a significant increase in OS when compared to IFN-α alone, perhaps due to the lower dose of temsirolimus administered in this group. Temsirolimus was generally well tolerated, with the most frequent grade 3–4 adverse events being asthenia, anaemia, and dyspnoea.

This study provided the key evidence for US FDA's approval of temsirolimus, and the European guidelines recommend temsirolimus as the first-line treatment in poor-risk patients with mRCC. In addition, patients with metastatic non-clear cell RCC instead of clear cell RCC appear to have a better survival benefit when treated with temsirolimus.

3.3.3.4 Pazopanib

Pazopanib is an oral multikinase angiogenesis inhibitor. It has received its European licence and will be marketed within the next few months. Whether it will be able to be used for NHS patients in the UK depends on the outcome of a review by NICE. A double-blind, randomized, placebo-controlled phase III study (n = 435) of pazopanib in treatment-naive and cytokine-pretreated patients with mRCC was presented at ASCO 2009. In this study, pazopanib exhibited impressive improvement in the primary outcome of PFS (9.2 months vs. 4.2 months) in the total population of treatment naïve and cytokine pretreated patients. PFS was 11.1 months in the treatment naïve population and 7.4 months in the cytokine pretreated population.

3.3.4 **Second-line treatment**

3.3.4.1 *Sorafenib*

Sorafenib is an oral tyrosine kinase inhibitor, which was originally developed as an inhibitor of Raf-1 (C-Raf), that is involved in the RAF/MEK/ERK signalling pathway. It was subsequently found to antagonize B-Raf, VEGF-2, VEGF-3, PDGF, Flt-3, and c-KIT.

A randomized phase III, double-blind, placebo-controlled trial of sorafenib (TARGET trial) in good- and intermediate-risk cytokine-refractory mRCC patients demonstrated a PFS and overall survival benefit for sorafenib after adjusting for crossover by censoring the placebo patients. Overall, treatment was generally well tolerated and these data led to the regulatory approval of sorafenib by the US FDA. Poor-risk patients, according to MSKCC criteria, were not included in this study and benefit-risk in these patients has not been evaluated.

A randomized phase II trial conducted to evaluate the effectiveness of sorafenib in the first-line setting compared to IFN-α in patients with metastatic disease failed to demonstrate a PFS benefit for sorafenib. The effectiveness of sorafenib as a first-line treatment in mRCC is unclear. Accordingly, the EMEA recommends sorafenib as a second-line agent in the treatment of mRCC post cytokine therapy.

Like sunitinib, sorafenib has an acceptable safety profile, with the majority of toxicities reported as mild to moderate. However, the main precautions to consider before starting a patient on sorafenib are summarized in Table 3.7.

- **Dermatological toxicities:** Hand–foot skin reaction (palmar-plantar erythrodysaesthesia) and rash represent the most common adverse drug reactions and generally appear during the first 6 weeks of treatment. Management of dermatological toxicities may include topical therapies for symptomatic relief, temporary treatment interruption in severe or persistent cases, and permanent discontinuation of sorafenib

- **Gastrointestinal perforation:** Gastrointestinal perforation has been reported in less than 1% of patients taking sorafenib, and it should be discontinued

- **Warfarin co-administration:** Infrequent bleeding events or elevations in international normalized ratio (INR) have been reported in some patients taking warfarin while on sorafenib therapy. Patients taking concomitant warfarin should be monitored regularly for changes in prothrombin time, INR, or clinical bleeding episodes

- **Elderly:** The experience with the use of sorafenib in elderly patients is limited but cases of renal failure have been reported. Renal function should be monitored.

Table 3.7 Precautions with sorafenib
Contraindications
• Paediatric use: safety and efficacy not established yet
• Hypersensitivity
• Severe uncontrolled hypertension (>200mmHg systolic or 110mmHg diastolic).
Cautions
• Cardiac events, pulmonary embolism, or cerebrovascular events
• Hepatic impairment—monitor as sorafenib eliminated via hepatic route
• Patients on anticoagulation.

Data from an ongoing multicentre, prospective phase II trial of sorafenib in patients with mRCC refractory to prior sunitinib or bevacizumab was presented at ASCO 2008. Tumour burden reduction rate (TBRR), the proportion of patients with >5% reduction in the sum of RECIST-defined target lesions without other progression, was 33% and 41% in patients with prior bevacizumab and sunitinib, respectively. The median PFS was 3.8 months. Several other small retrospective studies also suggest this lack of cross resistance and antitumour activity when VEGF-targeted agents are used in a sequential manner. This requires prospective investigation.

3.3.4.2 Everolimus (RAD001)

Everolimus is an orally administered mTOR inhibitor.

A randomized phase III trial compared everolimus with placebo in patients with good- or intermediate-risk features, as defined by MSKCC criteria, who had progressed on sunitinib or sorafenib therapy. The trial was stopped early following interim results analysis, which showed doubling of PFS (4 months vs. 2 months) in patients receiving everolimus compared to placebo.

On the basis of these results, the FDA has approved everolimus as a standard treatment of mRCC that have progressed on other targeted therapies.

References and further reading

Bellgrun AS (2007). Renal cell carcinoma: prognostic factors and patient selection. *European Urology Supplements*, **6**, 477–83.

Escudier B, Eisen T, Stadler WM, *et al.* (2007). Sorafenib in advanced clear-cell renal-cell carcinoma. *New England Journal of Medicine*, **356**, 125–34.

Escudier B, Pluzanska A, Koralewski P, *et al.* (2007). Bevacizumab plus interferon α for treatment of metastatic renal cell carcinoma: a randomised double blind phase III trial. *Lancet*, **370**, 2103–11.

European Association of Urology. Guidelines on renal cell carcinoma. Available at: http://www.uroweb.org/fileadmin/user_upload/Guidelines/Renal%20Cell%20Carcinoma.pdf. Accessed on 22nd June 2009.

Hudes G, Carducci M, Tomczak P, et al. (2007). Temsirolimus, interferon alfa, or both for advanced renal-cell carcinoma. *New England Journal of Medicine*, **356**, 2271–81.

Motzer RJ, Hutson TE, Tomczak P, et al. (2007). Sunitinib versus interferon-α in metastatic renal cell carcinoma. *New England Journal of Medicine*, **356**, 115–24.

National Comprehensive Guidelines Network. Kidney cancer. Available at: http://www.nccn.org/professionals/physician_gls/PDF/kidney.pdf. Accessed on 22nd June 2009.

Parton M, Gore M and Eisen T (2006). Role of cytokine therapy in 2006 and beyond for metastatic renal cell cancer. *Journal of Clinical Oncology*, **24**, 5584–92.

Rini B, Rathmell WK and Godley P (2008). Renal cell carcinoma. *Current Opinions in Oncology*, **20**, 300–6.

Samlowski WE, Wong B and Vogelzang NJ (2008). Management of renal cancer in the tyrosine kinase inhibitor era: a view from 3 years on. *British Journal of Urology International*, **102**, 162–5.

Chapter 4

The surgical approach

Arnaud Méjean and Marc-Olivier Timsit

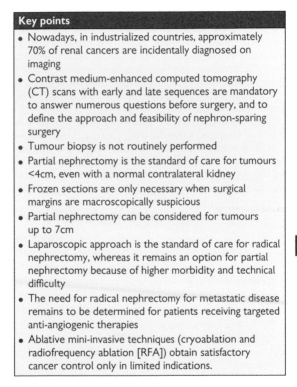

Key points

- Nowadays, in industrialized countries, approximately 70% of renal cancers are incidentally diagnosed on imaging
- Contrast medium-enhanced computed tomography (CT) scans with early and late sequences are mandatory to answer numerous questions before surgery, and to define the approach and feasibility of nephron-sparing surgery
- Tumour biopsy is not routinely performed
- Partial nephrectomy is the standard of care for tumours <4cm, even with a normal contralateral kidney
- Frozen sections are only necessary when surgical margins are macroscopically suspicious
- Partial nephrectomy can be considered for tumours up to 7cm
- Laparoscopic approach is the standard of care for radical nephrectomy, whereas it remains an option for partial nephrectomy because of higher morbidity and technical difficulty
- The need for radical nephrectomy for metastatic disease remains to be determined for patients receiving targeted anti-angiogenic therapies
- Ablative mini-invasive techniques (cryoablation and radiofrequency ablation [RFA]) obtain satisfactory cancer control only in limited indications.

4.1 Introduction

Surgical strategies to treat renal cell cancer (RCC) must meet the classical paradigm of cancer surgery: maximum chance of cure with minimal functional sequelae. Surgery has to be complete, leaving no residual tumour, while sparing as many nephrons as possible.

Performing conservative surgery without jeopardizing patients—the main objective—can be met when practitioners rigorously respect the following principles: identification of prognostic factors (evaluation of renal function and risk factors for renal failure) and meticulous imaging analysis (scrupulous procedure planning and stringent technical execution).

4.2 Presentation of RCC

Mean patient age at diagnosis is 64 years for sporadic RCC. Thus, if the patient's age is less than 45 years, complete physical examination and consideration of genetic testing are mandatory to screen for hereditary syndromes: von Hippel–Lindau disease, hereditary papillary RCC, hereditary leiomyomatosis and renal cell cancer (HLRCC) syndrome, Birt–Hogg–Dube syndrome, tuberous sclerosis, etc.

The main known risk factors of RCC are obesity, hypertension, and/or tobacco addiction.

Up to 70% of diagnoses are fortuitously made on imaging (ultrasonography or computed tomography [CT] scan) in asymptomatic patients.

In symptomatic patients, lumbar pain, haematuria, abdominal mass, hypertension, and varicocele are the classic presenting symptoms. Rarely, diagnosis is made on metastasis-related symptoms (seizure, respiratory disease, polyglobulia, inferior vena cava syndrome, etc.).

4.3 Required preoperative imaging

For all patients, thoracic and abdominal–pelvic CT scans are mandatory. The following questions must be answered before surgery:
- What is the size, volume, and location of the tumour?
- Is there a risk that the lesion could be a urothelial carcinoma?
- Is intratumour fat present (negative density on Hounsfield unit scale), specific to angiomyolipoma (non-malignant tumour)?
- Are imaging findings suggestive of renal oncocytoma (non-malignant), for example, a central scar?
- Is there evidence of macroscopic venous invasion (renal vein or vena cava)?
- Is there an evidence of spread beyond Gerota's fascia (T4 stage) meaning a risk of bowel invasion?
- Are there signs of metastatic disease?

Brain imaging or bone scintigraphy is needed only when abnormalities are detected during physical examination.

In the case of macroscopic venous invasion, vascular magnetic resonance imaging (MRI), and echocardiography are mandatory to evaluate the upper limit of the venous thrombus and anticipate the need for extracorporal circulation (or bypass) during surgery.

4.4 When should a renal lesion be biopsied?

This issue remains controversial among urologists. Indeed, the risk of the biopsy has to be balanced with the risk of removing a kidney bearing a benign tumour.

In all cases, the following rules must be strictly followed:
- Never biopsy a cystic lesion
- Never biopsy a suspected urothelial lesion
- Use a device with a retractable needle because of the theoretical risk of tract seeding
- A biopsy is essential in patients under 25 years old to look for a late nephroblastoma, which requires neoadjuvant chemotherapy
- Biopsy is required in patients with a prior cancer, especially a haematological malignancy (lymphoma).

On the basis of our experience, we recommend routine biopsy only in the following five common situations:
1. multifocal lesions suggestive of secondary lesions from another neoplasm;
2. imaging findings suggestive of a renal oncocytoma;
3. deep intrahilar tumour <4cm in diameter, as conservative surgery may be challenging and intraoperative difficulties may lead to radical nephrectomy;
4. past history of ipsi- or contralateral benign renal tumour;
5. prior ablative treatment (radiofrequency or cryoablation).

4.5 Surgical techniques and approaches

Since Robson's 1969 recommendation of radical nephrectomy and its subsequent rise to urology dogma, major concerns have arisen concerning renal function and risk of terminal renal failure. Thus, the concept of nephron-sparing surgery, initially developed for imperative indications (solitary kidney, end-stage renal disease, etc.), has been extended to relative and elective indications.

Table 4.1 lists the characteristics defining elective, relative, and imperative indications for partial nephrectomy, according to the cardinal principles of nephron-sparing surgery.

Renal function is often assessed with an estimation of glomerular filtration rate (eGFR). Although the wide differences can be calculated depending on the formula used (Cockroft–Gault vs. modification of diet in renal disease [MDRD] highlight), it is important to keep in mind the profound need for measured GFR (isotopic technique, iohexol clearance, etc.) in difficult cases to obtain a real idea of the patient's 'renal status' to anticipate the need for postoperative haemodialysis.

Table 4.1 Elective, relative, and absolute indications for partial nephrectomy

Partial nephrectomy indication	Contra-lateral kidney	Renal function	Risk of renal failure	Hereditary syndrome of papillary RCC
Elective	Normal	Normal	No	No
Relative	Small size or poorer relative function	Moderate renal insufficiency	Yes	No
Absolute	Absent	Advanced to severe renal failure	Any	Yes

Risk of disease recurrence is assessed according to prognostic scores (UISS [UCLA integrated staging system] or SSIGN [Mayo Clinic stage, size, grade, necrosis score]) based on TNM staging and other items (grade, presence of necrosis, and/or performance status) separating patients into low-, intermediate-, and high-risk groups with respective 5-year cancer-specific survival rates of 91%, 80%, and 55%.

According to preoperative clinical status and imaging, three situations are described as follows:

4.5.1 Localized tumours

4.5.1.1 RCC <4cm

Partial nephrectomy is recommended for tumours <4cm (pT1a), which have a 5-year progression-free survival rate of 95%. However, tumour location (centro-hilar) may render nephron-sparing surgery impracticable or increase the risk of incomplete resection; in these cases, a surgeon's skills and experience are determining factors.

The preferred approach is a lumbar incision; some authors recommend parenchymal clamping, when possible, to avoid vascular lesions and to procure a longer excision time without jeopardizing renal function (risk of extensive tubular necrosis).

In partial nephrectomy, the cardinal rules are as follows:

- Never let renal vascular clamping exceed 30 min without cooling
- Clamping (parenchymal or pedicular) is mandatory for a bloodless operating field to assure clear visibility to identify urinary ducts accurately and assess tumour extension

- Use scissors or scalpel (not electrocoagulation)
- The surgeon's macroscopic evaluation of surgical margins is accurate and useful (request frozen sections only when margins are doubtful)
- The thickness of safety margins is unimportant as long as they are negative.

Laparoscopic partial nephrectomy is feasible and achieved the same cancer control as open surgery, but may incur additional intra-operative and postoperative morbidity. Thus, at present, laparoscopy should continue to be considered as an optional approach, mainly for small exophytic masses (Figure 4.1). Because of its improved visibility and suturing facility, robotic assistance may have an expanding role in partial nephrectomy.

4.5.1.2 RCC <7cm

There is a current trend to extend the indications of partial nephrectomy (Figure 4.2) to tumours up to 7cm in diameter with elective indications, based on similar disease control compared with radical nephrectomy in all retrospective studies. Indeed, a recent study demonstrated that the risk of renal failure (MDRD <45mL/min) reached 45% 5 years after radical nephrectomy versus 7% after partial nephrectomy.

Still, careful patient selection is essential to limit morbidity and further prospective studies are needed to devise recommendations for tumours meeting elective indications.

For absolute indications, partial nephrectomy is mandatory to avoid terminal renal failure subsequent to radical nephrectomy and may be difficult for a tumour located deep in the hilum.

Ex vivo tumourectomy with renal self-transplantation may be an option but patients must be fully informed of the risk of kidney loss.

4.5.1.3 RCC >7cm (T2)

Radical nephrectomy is recommended for tumours >7cm in diameter, in a patient with a normal contralateral kidney (Figure 4.3). Because it is associated with less blood loss, fewer parietal complications, shorter hospital stays, and earlier returns to professional or daily activities than open radical nephrectomy, a laparoscopic approach is recommended and may soon be considered the gold standard of therapy for localized T2 tumours.

Once again, for imperative indications, the possibility of partial nephrectomy has to be considered. In some patients with many comorbidities, the risk of disease progression has to be counterbalanced with haemodialysis-associated morbidity.

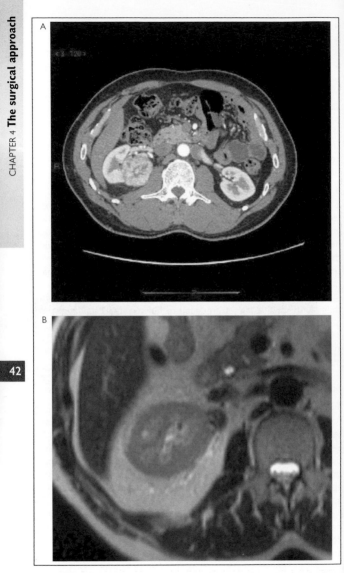

Figure 4.1 Nephron-sparing surgery and surgical approach: laparoscopic or lumbar incision for tumours in the right kidney? Partial nephrectomy is recommended for both patients but the approach will be different: open surgery and laparoscopic approach are, respectively, the best options for patients **A** (CT scan) and **B** (MRI).

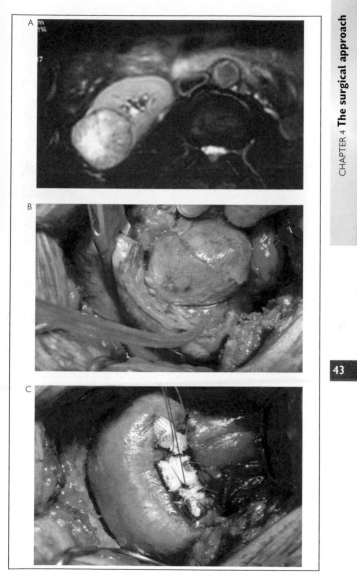

Figure 4.2 Nephron-sparing surgery. Partial nephrectomy of a 6-cm lesion (**A**) with a relative indication is performed with scissors under parenchymal clamping (**B**) and the remainder of the kidney is closed with sutures and resorbable haemostatic sponges (**C**).

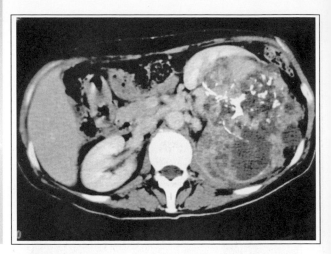

Figure 4.3 Laparoscopic surgery for locally advanced disease. Although voluminous on the CT scan, this RCC of the left kidney can be excised through a laparoscopic approach. However, in light of the risk of posterior muscle invasion and the technical difficulties resulting from the collateral venous circulation, patients must be informed preoperatively of the risk of an intraoperative switch to open surgery.

4.5.2 **Locally advanced RCC (renal vein and vena cava involvement T3b, T3c, N0, M0)**

Treatment consists of radical nephrectomy (Figure 4.4). Complete tumour thrombectomy is a major prognostic factor. Reported 5-year survival rates ranged from 25% to 70%.

When the suprahepatic inferior vena cava is involved by venous tumour extension, the surgical procedure might require extracorporal vascular bypass and sternotomy to allow right ventricular filling during clamping of the vena cava.

It is important to distinguish between a classical tumour thrombus (which is evacuated by cavotomy) and real tumour invasion of the vena cava wall that may require prosthetic replacement to ensure maximal resection.

Of course, in these cases, a laparoscopic approach is not feasible.

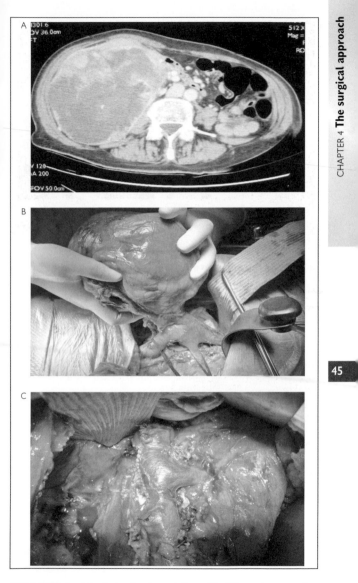

Figure 4.4 Open surgery for locally advanced disease. The CT scan shows a carcinoma of the right kidney with invasion of vena cava **(A)**. Surgical treatment requires complete ablation of the tumour thrombus **(B)** and suturing of the vena cava **(C)** at the end of the intervention.

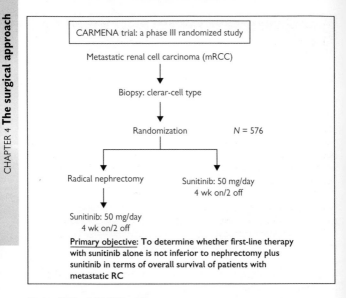

CARMENA trial: a phase III randomized study

Metastatic renal cell carcinoma (mRCC)

Biopsy: clerar-cell type

Randomization   N = 576

Radical nephrectomy   Sunitinib: 50 mg/day
                             4 wk on/2 off

Sunitinib: 50 mg/day
4 wk on/2 off

<u>Primary objective:</u> **To determine whether first-line therapy
with sunitinib alone is not inferior to nephrectomy plus
sunitinib in terms of overall survival of patients with
metastatic RC**

Figure 4.5 The CARMENA trial.

4.5.3 **Metastatic disease**

Primary radical nephrectomy remains the therapeutic gold standard. However, targeted and anti-angiogenic therapies have profoundly changed treatment options, raising numerous questions concerning the current standards of care. An ongoing European study (Figure 4.5: CARMENA trial) is trying to determine whether or not these (asymptomatic) patients require surgery, compared to targeted therapies alone (predominantly for the clear-cell subtype of RCC).

4.6 **Postoperative care**

Surgical complications are rarely observed after radical nephrectomy unless haemostasis was difficult to achieve intraoperatively. Complications of partial nephrectomy occur in 1% and 30% of patients, depending on the indications (respectively, elective and absolute), and mainly consist of haematoma, urinary fistula, and pseudoaneurysm. Their management includes endourological surgery or interventional radiology.

In the absence of complications and renal failure, patients are usually discharged on day 3 after laparoscopic surgery and day 5 after open surgery.

4.7 **Follow-up and surgery for relapsed disease**

4.7.1 **Adjuvant therapies**

At present, adjuvant treatment is not part of standard care.

4.7.2 **Ablative techniques**

Radiofrequency ablation and cryoablation, which use, respectively, electromagnetic waves generated by low-voltage alternating current, and extreme cooling through infusion and expansion of a refrigerant based on the Joule–Thompson effect, are two such techniques that achieve a satisfactory compromise among morbidity, nephron-sparing, and cancer control.

Indeed, they may be performed percutaneously, under local anaesthesia, without jeopardizing healthy peritumoural renal tissue. However, tumour size must be <3–5cm to assure complete destruction.

Thus, these techniques fulfil the requirement of minimal invasive treatment and should be considered excellent options in the following settings:

- Hereditary syndromes (von Hippel–Lindau, etc.), especially when tumours are <3cm
- History of multiple renal surgical procedures
- Solitary kidney, when tumour location renders partial nephrectomy difficult
- Advanced and end-stage renal disease
- Comorbid medical conditions contraindicating general anaesthesia
- Advanced age.

It is important to note that long-term follow-up of cancer control is not yet available and treatment efficacy may be difficult to assess. Therefore, partial nephrectomy should still be considered the best option when feasible.

When comparing recent series, cryoablation seems to be slightly superior to RFA in terms of tumour control, need for re-treatment, incidence of complications, and accuracy. Moreover, criteria of success during and after the procedures are more easily defined for cryoablation with the presence of an 'iceball' than for RFA because the contrast enhancement is more subjective and depends on the imaging technique (MRI, contrast-enhanced ultrasound, CT scan, etc.).

Concerning the risk of urinary leakage and pelvic retraction, RF should not be used for tumours that abut excretory ducts, at le not without endorenal cooling obtained through the use of a ure catheter to diffuse a cold saline solution during the procedure.

4.8 **Conclusion**

Tremendous modifications have been made over the past 10 years in the surgical approach to RCC. Urologists and oncologists are deeply concerned by the need for preservation of renal function and minimally invasive treatment. Notably, the arbitrary 4cm RCC threshold set for partial nephrectomy is rapidly giving way to calls for nephron-sparing surgery for even larger lesions.

Thus, the laparoscopic approach became a mandatory technique in the arsenal of surgeons dealing with these tumours, and robotic assistance must now prove its worth as a further improvement over laparoscopic partial nephrectomy.

Ablative treatments too seem to hold great promise for precise indications, mostly hereditary syndromes and medical comorbidities.

References and further reading

Cohen HT and McGovern FJ (2005). Renal-cell carcinoma. *New England Journal of Medicine*, **353(23)**, 2477–90.

Gill IS, Kavoussi LR, Lane BR, *et al*. (2007). Comparison of 1,800 laparoscopic and open partial nephrectomies for single renal tumors. *Journal of Urology*, **178(1)**, 41–6.

Huang WC, Levey AS, Serio AM, *et al*. (2006). Chronic kidney disease after nephrectomy in patients with renal cortical tumours: a retrospective cohort study. *Lancet Oncology*, **7(9)**, 735–40.

Patard JJ, Pantuck AJ, Crepel M, *et al*. (2007). Morbidity and clinical outcome of nephron-sparing surgery in relation to tumour size and indication. *European Urology*, **52(1)**, 148–54.

Timsit MO, Bazin JP, Thiounn N, *et al*. (2006). Prospective study of safety margins in partial nephrectomy: intraoperative assessment and contribution of frozen section analysis. *Urology*, **67(5)**, 923–6.

Uzzo RG and Novick AC (2001). Nephron sparing surgery for renal tumors: indications, techniques and outcomes. *Journal of Urology*, **166(1)**, 6–18.

Chapter 5

Interventional radiology

Khalid Enver and David Breen

Key points

- Percutaneous renal mass biopsy can aid in establishing a diagnosis, thus reducing the likelihood of unnecessary treatment for benign disease
- Small renal tumours can be successfully treated by image-guided ablation techniques, such as radio-frequency ablation and cryotherapy. Early follow-up data is promising
- Preoperative embolization can reduce the risk of complications from nephrectomy for renal cancer
- Embolization is also of benefit in the palliation of renal cancer and its metastases.

Interventional radiology plays a key role in the management of renal cancer. The interventional radiologist may contribute to the diagnosis of a renal mass by performing a biopsy or treating a renal mass or its metastases by ablation or embolization.

5.1 Diagnosis

5.1.1 Renal biopsy

The increased use of abdominal imaging has led to the increased detection of incidental renal lesions. The majority of these are simple cysts that are benign. However, solid or complex cystic renal masses can be malignant, and it can be difficult to establish a diagnosis on imaging characteristics alone. Small lesions are also much more likely to be benign, with benign histology found in 25% of resected tumours smaller than 3cm and almost half of all tumours <1cm.

There is a role for biopsy, particularly in small volume renal masses, to better identifying malignant disease, thus avoiding unnec-essary treatment for benign disease. Limitations in biopsy have been identified; for example, a study of biopsies performed on excised masses at the time of nephrectomy found 20% of returns to be non-diagnostic, and the sensitivity for identifying malignancy of only 81%. However, there are recent studies of image-guided biopsy, in which as few as 4% of specimens are non-diagnostic, and the sensitivity for the detection of malignancy is up to 98%. Biopsy is also useful in differentiating renal cell carcinoma (RCC) from renal lymphoma, metastases and abscess, and in providing a histological diagnosis in patients with a renal mass who are not surgical candidates.

5.1.2 **Biopsy technique**

The patient is consented, and clotting parameters are checked. In our institute, the vast majority of biopsies are performed under ultrasound guidance. The patient is positioned appropriately to allow best access, usually in the lateral, oblique, or prone position. The lesion is examined in several planes, and note made of cystic or necrotic components that may limit diagnostic yield. Local anaesthetic is infiltrated at the skin entry site and into the abdominal wall. Care is taken to avoid injecting air bubbles that may obscure the lesion. A 16G or 18G cutting core biopsy needle is inserted under real-time ultrasound guidance. Breathing is suspended when the needle is to be advanced into the kidney, and as the device is fired. Two cores are usually obtained, and the specimens are placed in formalin. The patient is then rescanned to check for post-biopsy haemorrhage and closely observed for 4hr.

A haematoma may be identified on computed tomography (CT) in 91% of post-renal biopsy patients. However, clinically significant haemorrhage is only noted in <1% of post-biopsy patients. Pseudoaneurysm and arteriovenous fistula are recognized delayed complications in <1% of biopsies, which may present with retroperitoneal haemorrhage. Seeding along the biopsy track is rare, with an estimated incidence of 1 in 20,000.

5.1.3 **Diagnostic angiography**

Advances in non-invasive imaging have led to the abandonment of angiography in the diagnosis of renal tumours.

5.2 **Ablation therapy**

Tumour ablation can be achieved in smaller renal tumours, usually <4cm, by percutaneous ablation therapies such as radiofrequency ablation (RFA) and cryotherapy, which induce thermal necrosis within the tumour. The treated tumours remain in situ, rather than resected as in surgery.

5.2.1 **Ablation**

Image-guided ablation (IGA) offers benefits when compared to surgery. There is lower morbidity and mortality, the costs are lower, and patients who are high-risk surgical candidates can usually be treated. The treatments are nephron sparing, thus minimizing the long-term morbidity of additional renal impairment, and reducing the risk of renal replacement therapy. The procedure involves placing one or more thin probes, under image guidance, into the renal lesion. Thermal energy is applied for adequate time to ensure necrosis within not only the tumour, but also within a substantial margin of normal renal tissue at its periphery, to ensure adequate ablation of the tumour margin. Procedural variables such as probe choice, device settings, and treatment time must be adjusted to ensure certainty about the volume and adequacy of the ablation treatment. Follow-up imaging needs to confirm treatment of tumour, usually by means of non-enhancement at post-contrast imaging, and also monitor for local recurrence, new tumours or metastases. RFA and cryotherapy have emerged as the main techniques for IGA for renal tumours. The use of other thermal ablative techniques, such as microwave and high-intensity focused ultrasound, are developing.

There are tumours, particularly small lesions, which are not visible on ultrasound or unenhanced CT, and can only be identified for a short period on enhanced CT imaging. Placing of the tip is then coordinate guided, rather than image guided. In these cases, it is important to ensure that the patient is still on the CT scanner, and that adjustments are made to compensate for renal respiratory movement. The use of fused CT and ultrasound imaging has been shown to further aid image guidance. Magnetic resonance (MR)-guided ablation is practised, but is technically easiest with an open system or a wide bore conventional closed bore system. Equipment needs to be MR compatible, with issues typically related to electrical interference, image degradation, and device heating.

5.2.2 **Radiofrequency ablation**

In monopolar RFA, a high frequency (400–500kHz) alternating current is applied to the patient. The current passes from the tiny RFA probe tip to a large grounding pad on the patient, with the patient forming part of the electrical circuit. Frictional heating occurs as a result of ion agitation at the probe tip, where the current density and heat concentration is high, with heat conducted into the adjacent target tissues.

Coagulative necrosis can occur at temperatures as low as 46°C, but cell death can take up to 1hr. Cell death is instantaneous at above 60°C. Above 105°C tissue boils, vaporizes, and carbonizes, but this may impair heat propagation through the target lesion. Therefore, the aim of RFA treatment is to induce coagulative necrosis by maintaining a temperature of between 60°C and 105°C throughout the entire target volume. Current RFA devices create a 3–5cm sphere of ablated tissue within a practical time frame.

Patients are selected for image-guided ablation following multidisciplinary team discussion. After disease staging, patients are preassessed to determine the optimum imaging modality and approach for ablation, and their suitability for conscious sedation or general anaesthesia. Ablation may be performed under CT, ultrasound or MR guidance, or a combination of modalities.

Several RFA probes are available. Some comprise multiple expandable tines, projecting from the tip of a 14G or 15G needle-like probe. The tines can be extended into the target lesion at 1cm increments to suit the desired treatment volume. Other probes consist of a 17G needle or a cluster of three needles in a triangular configuration.

Needle biopsy can be performed before, or at the time of ablation, according to multidisciplinary management discussion. An average treatment time for a 3cm tumour would be 20 min, aiming for a mean target temperature of 105°C throughout the tumour volume. Most operators advocate 'track ablation' at the end of the procedure to reduce the potential risk of track seeding.

5.2.3 Cryotherapy

Cryotherapy (from the Greek 'kruos' meaning icy cold) is therapeutic *in situ* tissue destruction by freezing. Its use had been limited to open surgical procedures because of a large probe size, but the development of narrow gauge argon probes has enabled treatment via a percutaneous approach. Low temperatures are achieved by the rapid conversion of a high pressure inert gas into a low pressure liquid. The temperature at the argon probe tip is −150°C, typically creating a 2cm ice ball, largely at less than −20°C throughout, which causes tissue destruction when at least two freeze-thaw cycles are applied. Cell death occurs from protein damage as the cell dehydrates in response to freezing, damaging the cell membrane and intracellular enzymes. The formation of ice crystals within the cell also damages intracellular organelles and the cell membrane.

The use of multiple adjacent probes can allow sculpting of the ice ball shape and size, thus allowing larger treatment zones. Three parallel probes are typically required to treat a 3cm lesion. Cell death in the ice ball is maximized by rapid cooling to less than −40°C, with multiple freeze-thaw cycles. The ice ball has characteristic appearances on imaging. On ultrasound it is a highly echogenic structure with posterior acoustic shadowing. On CT and magnetic resonance imaging (MRI), the cryoablation treatment zone is clearly demonstrated, with crisp demarcation from adjacent tissues.

5.2.4 **Follow-up after ablation**

As the tumour is treated in situ rather than resected, follow-up imaging is essential. Initial imaging within the first 2 weeks is to assess adequacy of treatment, as the zone of absolute tissue death is best defined at least a few days post-procedure. Further regular follow-up is to monitor for local recurrence or metastatic disease. CT is the most commonly used modality for follow-up imaging, but in cases where intravenous contrast cannot be given, follow-up by MR or contrast-enhanced ultrasound is performed. There is a lack of consensus about the optimum frequency and duration of surveillance, but in our institute imaging is performed at 6 monthly intervals to 2 years and then annually to 5 years.

Lack of enhancement within the tumour is considered a surrogate for tumour ablation. At our institute, late arterial phase and portal venous phase follow-up CT imaging is performed. The absence of tumour enhancement, growth, and gradual lesion involution are indicators of successful treatment. A slender ablation 'halo' is often noted in the perinephric fat surrounding a successfully treated lesion. On follow-up of over 5 years, our experience has been that lesions completely resolve, leaving only a small cortical scar, or reduce to a small volume of non-enhancing tissue, as shown in Figure 5.1. MR follow-up is also possible, with contrast subtraction techniques useful in those with a contraindication to CT contrast agents. Post-procedure biopsy has been found to be a poor determinant of treatment adequacy, as the dead tumour cells often appear structurally intact, but in fact are not viable when examined using tissue viability stains.

Nephron-sparing techniques, such as IGA, are often undertaken in patients with significant renal impairment. The risk of contrast-induced nephropathy needs to be taken into account when performing contrast-enhanced CT studies in these patients. Iso- or low-osmolality contrast agents, as well as prehydration, can minimize the risk of contrast induced nephropathy (CIN). MR contrast imaging is also affected by renal impairment, with patients at risk of nephrogenic systemic fibrosis (NSF). It is believed that free Gd^{3+} contributes to NSF and that risk of NSF may be reduced by the use of macrocyclic chelating agents rather than linear gadolinium agents, as these molecules are less likely to dissociate Gd^{3+}.

5.2.5 **Outcomes**

There are several published single and multi-institutional case series. There are no randomized trials comparing the outcome of image-guided ablation and surgery.

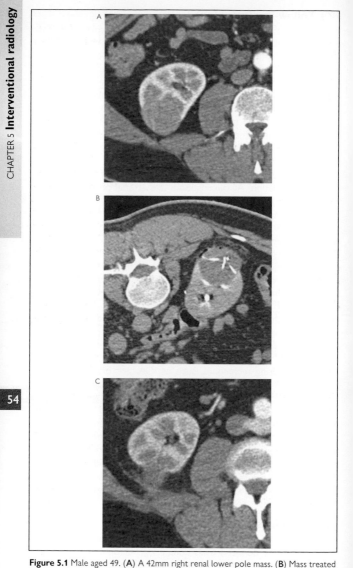

Figure 5.1 Male aged 49. (**A**) A 42mm right renal lower pole mass. (**B**) Mass treated by CT-guided RFA with patient prone. Tip of RF probe and tines demonstrated within lesion. Biopsy at procedure confirmed RCC. (**C**) Eight months post-treatment successfully treated unenhancing RF lesion continues to involute, now measuring only 25mm.

Sixty-nine to ninety-seven per cent of tumours are successfully treated completely at a single setting (5–10). The rates are better in centres that treat smaller tumours, as it tends to be larger tumours that require re-treatment. Ninety-seven to hundred per cent of tumours <3.5cm are completely ablated at a single setting. The management of patients with residual disease after their first ablation therapy may vary. At our centre, in a cohort of 97 patients with 105 relatively large tumours (mean 3.2cm), 79% of tumours were completely ablated at the first treatment session. Of the 22 tumours with residual disease, following multidisciplinary discussion, 7 were managed conservatively with interval imaging, 1 had a nephrectomy, and 15 proceeded to repeat ablation. Only two patients were left with residual disease after repeated ablation treatment, one of which was because of a pneumothorax that led to procedure abandonment.

Long-term post-RFA follow-up study data are typically limited to a mean of only a few years. The two studies with longest follow-up have a mean follow-up of 61 months in 31 patients and 55 months in 19 patients, respectively. In these studies, local disease recurrence is found in 6–10%. Metastasis free and disease-specific survival is 100%. Local recurrence may represent residual microscopic cancer that has become grossly detectable on follow-up imaging. However, the numbers of patients in these studies are small, and there is a large volume of follow-up data that will be available in the next few years.

Long-term cryotherapy studies are from treatment at open or laparoscopic procedures rather than percutaneous treatment. The study with longest follow-up, in 48 patients with median follow-up of 64 months, found that 12.5% of patients had residual tumour after initial treatment, but only 3% after subsequent ablation sessions. Eight per cent were found to have disease recurrence beyond 12 months. Metastases were found in a single patient, but there was a cancer-specific survival rate of 100%. A meta-analysis of small renal mass treatment outcomes from 47 RFA and cryotherapy case series found cryotherapy initial treatment failure rates to be lower than those of RFA (1.3% vs. 8.5%).

Major complication rates are <5% for percutaneous cryotherapy and RFA. Techniques such as hydrodissection, in which 250–750mL of 5% dextrose are instilled into the retroperitoneum around the tumour to create a safety margin by displacing adjacent structures, helps to minimize local complications from thermal injury.

The preliminary data are promising and suggest that ablation therapies will play a significant role in the treatment of small volume renal tumours in the future.

5.3 **Embolization therapy**

5.3.1 **Embolization before surgery**

In the absence of a randomized study, the survival benefits of transarterial embolization (TAE) are unclear. A case matched study of stage T2, T3, and T3 with lymphadenopathy renal carcinoma found a survival benefit when nephrectomy was combined with preoperative embolization, compared to nephrectomy alone. The reasons for this survival benefit are unclear, but may involve immune modulation from tumour ischaemic necrosis as a result of the embolization. However, several other studies have not identified a survival benefit from preoperative embolization.

Preoperative embolization is thought to minimize blood loss, reduce tumour bulk, and ease tumour dissection in nephrectomy of large renal masses with extensive collateral vasculature, as shown in Figure 5.2. There is evidence that blood transfusion requirements at nephrectomy are reduced by preoperative embolization, although operating time is not affected.

Embolization can also reduce the extent and size of tumour thrombus in patients with tumour extending into the renal vein and inferior vena cava, although there is a described risk of tumour embolization. At surgery, the renal artery is usually ligated before the renal vein, but this may not be possible because of hilar nodes or perihilar disease. Preoperative TAE can allow operative ligation of the renal vein first.

Embolization agents include metallic microcoils, acrylic microspheres, polvinyl alcohol particles, absolute ethanol, and gelfoam. Patients may suffer from post-infarction syndrome, and have severe pain, nausea, and vomiting. The ideal time for surgery after TAE is at 48–72 hr, as there is some evidence that the plane between the tumour and renal bed is easiest to dissect at this stage.

5.3.2 **Palliative therapy**

There is an accepted role for embolization in the modulation of symptoms from advanced RCC, including control of haematuria, pain, polycythaemia, hypercalcaemia, hypertension, and cardiac failure. There is little evidence to suggest a survival benefit from TAE. Repeated embolization is often needed to control symptoms, but becomes increasingly difficult as a result of tumour vascular parasitization from lumbar and mesenteric vessels.

Forty per cent of RCC patients will at some stage develop bony metastases, and RCC is the fourth commonest metastatic tumour to affect the spine. Malignant infiltration of the spine can cause pain, radiculopathy, and cord compression. The metastases from RCC are hypervascular, as shown in Figure 5.3, and there is a significantly increased risk of perioperative blood loss associated with surgery.

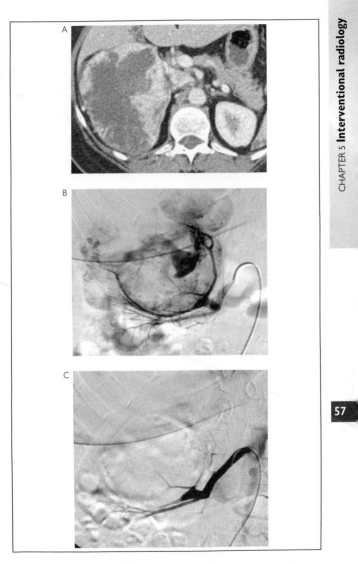

Figure 5.2 Female aged 61. (**A**) A 12cm mass centred on the upper pole of the right kidney. (**B**) Renal artery angiography shows a large hypervascular mass with a grossly abnormal arteriovenous shunt and large vascular pool. (**C**) Gelatin sponge (Spongistan gelfoam) and subsequent spherical polyvinyl alcohol (PVA) hydrogel (Bead Block) used to embolize renal artery, with stasis achieved in the renal artery on post-treatment angiogram. (Images courtesy of Dr N Hacking.)

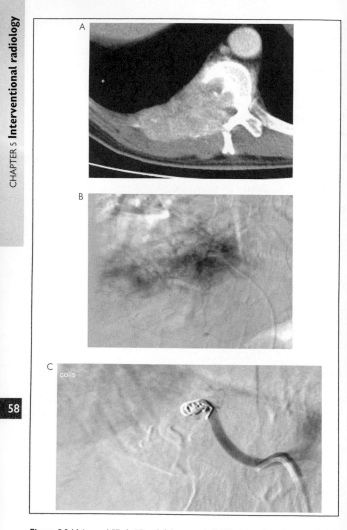

58

Figure 5.3 Male aged 57. A 4.5cm left lower pole RCC with multiple bone metastases. Radicular pain of D10. (**A**) Large metastasis centred on the right side of D10 vertebra, which extends into the pedicle, neural arch, and hemibody of D10. (**B**) Selective catheterization of D10 lumbar artery demonstrates the hypervascular D10 vertebral metastasis. The tumour blood supply originates from the right D9 and D10 lumbar arteries. (**C**) Selective catheterization of the D9 lumbar and D10 lumbar vertebrae with occlusion by microcoils. Post-procedure angiogram of D10 lumbar artery confirms satisfactory tumour devascularization. (Images courtesy of Dr N Hacking.)

Spinal surgeons consider embolization essential before surgical decompression and spinal fixation in these patients. Selective bilateral angiograms of segmental intercostal or lumbar arteries to cover a region two levels above and below the affected vertebra are performed. To avoid non-target embolization of intercostal or lumbar arteries, the arteries distal to the origins of tumour feeders are occluded with platinum microcoils. Embolization of bone metastases can also be performed for symptom relief, without surgery, and is also performed elsewhere in the skeleton, most commonly in the femur and humerus. Interventional radiology techniques can similarly provide palliative management through percutaneous vertebroplasty.

References and further reading

Breen DJ, Rutherford EE, Stedman B, et al. (2007). Management of renal tumors by image-guided radiofrequency ablation: experience in 105 tumors. *Cardiovascular and Interventional Radiology*, **30(5)**, 936–42.

Davol PE, Fulmer BR and Rukstalis DB (2006). Long-term results of cryoablation for renal cancer and complex renal masses. *Urology*, **68(1 Suppl)**, 2–6.

Dechet CB, Zincke H, Sebo TJ, et al. (2003). Prospective analysis of computerized tomography and needle biopsy with permanent sectioning to determine the nature of solid renal masses in adults. *Journal of Urology*, **169(1)**, 71–4.

Frank I, Blute ML, Cheville JC, Lohse CM, Weaver AL and Zincke H (2003). Solid renal tumors: an analysis of pathological features related to tumor size. *Journal of Urology*, **170(6 Pt 1)**, 2217–20.

Kunkle DA and Uzzo RG (2008). Cryoablation or radiofrequency ablation of the small renal mass: a meta-analysis. *Cancer*, **113(10)**, 2671–80.

Levinson AW, Su LM, Agarwal D, et al. (2008). Long-term oncological and overall outcomes of percutaneous radio frequency ablation in high risk surgical patients with a solitary small renal mass. *Journal of Urology*, **180(2)**, 499–504.

Matin SF, Ahrar K, Cadeddu JA, et al. (2006). Residual and recurrent disease following renal energy ablative therapy: a multi-institutional study. *Journal of Urology*, **176(5)**, 1973–7.

Maturen KE, Nghiem HV, Caoili EM, Higgins EG, Wolf JS Jr and Wood DP Jr (2007). Renal mass core biopsy: accuracy and impact on clinical management. *American Journal of Roentgenology*, **188(2)**, 563–70.

McDougal WS, Gervais DA, McGovern FJ and Mueller PR (2005). Long-term followup of patients with renal cell carcinoma treated with radiofrequency ablation with curative intent. *The Journal of Urology*, **174(1)**, 61–3.

Silverman SG, Israel GM, Herts BR and Richie JP (2008). Management of the incidental renal mass. *Radiology*, **249(1)**, 16–31.

Zagoria RJ, Traver MA, Werle DM, Perini M, Hayasaka S and Clark PE (2007). Oncologic efficacy of CT-guided percutaneous radiofrequency ablation of renal cell carcinomas. *American Journal of Roentgenology*, **189(2)**, 429–36.

Zielinski H, Szmigielski S and Petrovich Z (2000). Comparison of preoperative embolization followed by radical nephrectomy with radical nephrectomy alone for renal cell carcinoma. *American Journal of Clinical Oncology*, **23(1)**, 6–12.

Chapter 6

Systemic treatment: immunotherapy

Bernard Escudier, Marine Gross Goupil,
Christophe Massard, and Karim Fizazi

Key points

- For 20 years, immunotherapy has been the standard of care for renal cell carcinoma (RCC)
- Although the new targeted therapies have dramatically changed the landscape of this disease, immunotherapy remains an attractive therapeutic option in this disease
- Initially, there have been two main reasons for developing immunotherapy in RCC
  - The resistance to any kind of chemotherapy
  - The observation that spontaneous remission was observed in this disease, strongly suggesting the role of immune system
- The enthusiasm for immunotherapy was then greatly stimulated by the initial results of high-dose interleukin 2 (IL-2), demonstrating a significant proportion of patients achieving partial or even complete remission, with sustained responses and long-lasting responses. Furthermore, the first results with the use of interferon (IFN) confirmed that responses could be observed with cytokines
- These exciting data stimulated research in the field of immunology and immunotherapy of RCC, and led to the attempt to treat the disease with different types of immune manipulations, including cell therapy, vaccines, and bone marrow transplantation.

The aim of this review is to give an overview of the current status of immunotherapy in renal cell carcinoma (RCC), both as an adjuvant therapy for non-metastatic disease and as a treatment of more advanced disease.

6.1 Immunotherapy as adjuvant treatment in RCC (Table 6.1)

6.1.1 Cytokines

On the basis of the activity of interleukin 2 (IL-2) and interferon (IFN) on metastatic disease, several studies have tried to demonstrate the activity of cytokines in the adjuvant setting. It is fair to say that many large studies have been performed, and that none of them have been able to demonstrate any benefit.

Because of the ease of using IFN, most of the studies have tested IFN in RCC patients at risk of relapse. Three studies have been reported with different schedules of IFN, with 88–283 patients enrolled depending on the study, and no benefit in terms of disease-free survival (DFS) or overall survival.

High-dose IL-2 has also been evaluated in a single randomized trial of 44 patients. DFS was not different and the trial was stopped because of toxicity and very low likelihood that a larger trial would provide advantage to IL-2.

Combination of IL-2 and IFN has also been tested. In a German study comparing this combination to the observation in 203 patients, no benefit was observed. More recently, the preliminary results of a larger study from EORTC on 309 patients randomized between a triple combination of IL-2, IFN, and 5-fluorouracil (5FU) were reported with no benefit for the regimen in terms of disease free or overall survival.

All together, these studies, although often underpowered to demonstrate significant benefit, do not encourage further investigation of adjuvant cytokine therapy in RCC.

Study	Cytokine regimen	Number of patients	DFS treatment group (%)	DFS observation group (%)
Gotoh, 2004	sc IFN	88	81	–
Pizzocaro, 2001	sc IFN	247	56.7	67.1
Messing, 2003	sc IFN	283	37	41
Clark, 2003	High-dose IL-2	44	23.8	34.8
Atzpodien, 2005	IFN+IL-2+5FU	203	42	49

Table 6.1 Efficacy of cytokines in adjuvant setting (5-year DFS results)

6.1.2 **Vaccines and antibodies**

Despite the lack of common antigens in RCC, different approaches of vaccine therapy have been tested in the adjuvant setting: autologous tumour vaccines and heat shock proteins (HSPs) have been recently reported in large randomized trials.

6.1.2.1 *Tumour cell lysate vaccines*

The hypothesis that tumour cell lysates contain tumour antigens has been used to develop this approach in RCC. A large randomized phase III trial was reported in 2004 using an autologous vaccine injected intradermally. Although the trial showed a significant benefit in DFS, multiple potential biases including a large number of patients who could not receive the vaccine, have made these results controversial. Later, an update of the trial found a statistical improvement in DFS in the vaccine group compared to an observation in an intent-to-treat analysis, highlighting the need to pursue such approaches in the future with a statistically robust trial design.

6.1.2.2 *Heat shock proteins*

These proteins represent a major class of chaperone proteins which play a crucial role in antigen presentation. HSPs such as HSP 96 have demonstrated activity in *in vivo* models and further in metastatic RCC. This rationale was the basis for a large phase III trial in 816 patients with non-metastatic RCC. The final results of this study have been recently published. Although this study failed to reach its endpoint of improving DFS in an intent-to-treat analysis, exploratory analyses by tumour stage demonstrated positive RFS and OS trends associated with vaccination among patients with T1 + T2 disease ($n = 251$) and T3a disease ($n = 191$). On the basis of this trend, approval for this vaccine has been obtained in Russia, and is currently under review at the European Medicines Evaluation Agency (EMEA).

6.1.2.3 *G250 antibody*

This antibody, also named carbonic anhydrase IX (CA IX), was identified as a RCC-associated antigen absent in normal kidney and homogeneously expressed in clear cell RCC. On the basis of the favourable tissue distribution, pilot phase I and II studies were performed in metastatic RCC, with some signal of activity. On the basis of these results, a large multicentre study has been performed to assess the activity of this antibody versus placebo in adjuvant setting. Enrolment for this phase III has been completed, and results are expected in the next 2–5 years.

Overall, adjuvant treatment of RCC with immunotherapy remains interesting although all the reported studies have failed so far to confirm the benefit. Currently, there is more enthusiasm for targeted therapies in this setting based on efficacy of VEGF-targeted therapies in metastatic RCC, and large trials are ongoing with either sorafenib or sunitinib in high- and intermediate-risk non-metastatic RCC.

6.2 **Immunotherapy in metastatic RCC**

6.2.1 **Cytokines**

IL-2 and IFN have been the standard of care for patients with metastatic RCC until very recently. Despite the use of these agents for more than 20 years, the efficacy of these two drugs is still controversial.

Several important studies have defined the utility of immunotherapy in RCC.

Bolus high-dose intravenous IL-2 treatment initially generated great enthusiasm, yet subsequent randomized trials failed to demonstrate a benefit over lower-dose cytokine regimens. Most important, however, durable complete remissions occur in 5–10% of patients, distinguishing this therapy and serving as the basis for FDA approval in the United States. Thus, despite the associated toxicity of capillary leak syndrome, IL-2 remains a viable treatment option reserved for patients with a good performance status and acceptable comorbid conditions. Current investigative efforts include attempts to identify the molecular phenotype of response to IL-2 to maximize benefit. Recent results show that high expression of a von Hippel–Landau (VHL)-mediated protein called CA IX may predict for response to IL-2. There are also pathological features of the primary renal tumour which may further help determine those patients who are likely to benefit from IL-2. A specific study aiming to validate these predictive factors of response is ongoing in the United States.

Two large randomized trials have demonstrated that IFN improves survival when compared with medroxyprogesterone acetate (MPA) or vinblastine. A Cochrane review also supports the use of IFN. On the basis of these studies, IFN monotherapy became the standard comparator for the evaluation of new treatments in metastatic RCC until the TKI era.

Combining low-dose IL-2 and IFN together improves response rates and progression-free survival (PFS) over either as monotherapy, but overall survival is not improved with combination therapy. Further, switching to the other cytokine after failure on either cytokine is not useful. Whether this combination should be better by using intravenous IL-2 has also been explored by the French group, but their study failed to detect any difference between intravenous and subcutaneous IL-2.

The role of IL-2 and IFN has been further studied in an intermediate prognostic group of patients. These cytokines failed to demonstrate a PFS or OS benefit over MPA. This study highlights the fact that, as with high-dose IL-2, stringent patient selection efforts are warranted. Identification of clinical and/or biological predictors of response to these cytokines remains an area of active investigation.

As noted earlier the addition of chemotherapy to cytokine regimens, despite initial reports of high response rates and benefits in small randomized trials, did not show definitive benefits over cytokine monotherapy when subjected to a large randomized comparison.

In summary, these studies demonstrate a modest benefit of cytokine monotherapy in unselected cohorts, and suggest that the greatest benefit is achieved when applied to a very select, good prognosis patient group, potentially achieving durable remissions. The role of cytokines in the current era of metastatic RCC should be restricted as such, in addition to proven combination regimens with targeted therapy. Additional cytokine combination regimens and patient selection efforts remain an area of active investigation.

6.2.2 **Other immunotherapy**

On the basis of the relative efficacy of cytokines, various immunotherapeutic approaches have been tested in RCC.

6.2.2.1 Cell therapy

An attempt to improve the efficacy of IL-2 was made in the late 1980s by using T cells in addition to IL-2. Different approaches were used, including LAK cells (lymphokine-activated killer cells), NK (natural killer) cells, or TILs (tumour-infiltrating cells). All these studies, although encouraging were discouraged by the results of a randomized phase III study of CD8 TILs selected from the primary tumour, in 178 patients, which was negative.

6.2.2.2 Dendritic cell vaccination

Dendritic cells (DCs) are very potent antigen-presenting cells, which play an important role in the control of immunity. Immature and mature DCs have been loaded with peptide, recombinant protein, whole tumour lysates, mRNA, etc., and different routes of administration have been studied (intravenous, intradermal, subcutaneous, intralymphatic, etc.). Thus far, more than 200 patients with metastatic RCC have been treated with DC vaccination. Following very exciting preliminary results with a German vaccine, prepared with allogeneic DC fused with autologous tumour cells, this approach has been widely tested in the early 2000s. Unfortunately, the initial manuscript was further withdrawn, and enthusiasm rapidly decreased with the failure to reproduce objective responses in metastatic RCC.

However, DC vaccination can induce tumour-specific T-cell responses and thus remains a potential field of exploration.

6.2.2.3 Allogeneic stem cell transplantation

On the basis of the hypothesis that donor CD8+ cytotoxic T lymphocytes recognize minor histocompatibility antigens on recipient tissues, and can induce graft-versus-tumour effects, non-myeloablative allogeneic cell transplantation has been initiated in solid tumours. After initial case reports of successful treatment with this approach in metastatic RCC, the initial study from Childs et al. generated great enthusiasm. In 19 patients with progressive metastases after high-dose IL-2, allogeneic bone marrow transplantation-induced objective clinical response in 10 patients (53%), with 3 patients (16%) reaching complete remission. Subsequent studies have confirmed that similar treatment could induce objective responses, but with a lower magnitude and a high incidence of treatment-related complications and mortality. Owing to this high toxicity and the development of new targeted therapies, the real benefit of this technique will be difficult to study in future prospective trials.

6.2.2.4 Various vaccine and monoclonal antibody therapies

Different approaches, such as HSPs and monoclonal antibody therapy with G250, have been tested in metastatic RCC. Although some signal of activity has been reported in phase I–II, none of these studies were convincing enough to encourage the development of these treatments in metastatic RCC. However, these results led to phase III trials in the adjuvant setting as reported earlier. The phase III study of HSP 96 failed to improve DFS in the intent-to-treat analysis, and the G250 trial is ongoing. If this trial does turn out to be positive, targeted immunotherapy would probably become a new opportunity in RCC. Apart from these treatments, monoclonal antibody against VEGF (bevacizumab) has demonstrated clinical activity both in phase II and in phase III in metastatic RCC. However, this treatment is mainly active through its antiangiogenic activity and will be described extensively in chapter 7.

In conclusion, immunotherapy with cytokines and other more sophisticated approaches generated great enthusiasm in the 1990s, but further large studies have shown that the benefit was restricted to a highly selected patient population. Better selection of the patients and/or new targeted immunotherapy could help to define those patients who should continue to be treated with cytokines, and whether immunotherapy could continue to play a role in the treatment of RCC. The observation that long lasting complete remissions can occur with high-dose IL-2, for example, still constitutes a rationale to develop effective immunotherapy in this disease.

References and further reading

Aitchison M, Bray C, Van Poppel H, et al. (2008). Preliminary results from a randomized phase III trial of adjuvant interleukin-2, interferon alpha and 5-fluorouracil in patients with a high risk of relapse after nephrectomy for renal cell carcinoma (RCC). Journal of Clinical Oncology, 26(Suppl), abstract 5040.

Assikis VJ, Daliani D, Pagliaro L, et al. (2003). Phase II study of an autologous tumor derived heat shock protein-peptide complex vaccine (HSPPC-96) for patients with metastatic renal cell carcinoma (mRCC) [abstract]. Proceedings of the American Society of Clinical Oncology, 22, 386 (abstract 1552).

Atkins M, Regan M, McDermott D, et al. (2005). Carbonic anhydrase IX expression predicts outcome of interleukin 2 therapy for renal cancer. Clinical Cancer Research, 11(10), 3714–21.

Atzpodien J, Kirchner H, Hanninen EL, Deckert M, Fenner M and Poliwoda H (1993). Interleukin-2 in combination with interferon-alpha and 5-fluorouracil for metastatic renal cell cancer. European Journal of Cancer, 29A(Suppl 5), S6–8.

Atzpodien J, Kirchner H, Illiger HJ, et al. (2001). IL-2 in combination with IFN-alpha and 5-FU versus tamoxifen in metastatic renal cell carcinoma: long-term results of a controlled randomized clinical trial. British Journal of Cancer, 85(8), 1130–6.

Atzpodien J, Kirchner H, Jonas U, et al. (2004). Interleukin-2- and interferon alfa-2a-based immunochemotherapy in advanced renal cell carcinoma: a Prospectively Randomized Trial of the German Cooperative Renal Carcinoma Chemoimmunotherapy Group (DGCIN). Journal of Clinical Oncology, 22(7), 1188–94.

Atzpodien J, Kirchner H, Illiger HJ, et al. (2005). Interleukin-2 and IFN alfa-2a based chemoimmunotherapy in RCC post tumor nephrectomy: results of a prospectively randomized trial of the German Co-operative Renal Carcinoma Chemoimmunotherapy Group (DGCIN). British Journal of Cancer, 92, 843–6.

Banchereau J and Steinman RM (1998). Dendritic cells and the control of immunity. Nature, 392, 245–52.

Bernsten A, Geertsen PF and Svane IM (2006). Therapeutic dendritic cell vaccination of patients with RCC. European Urology, 50, 34–43.

Bleumer I, Knuth A, Oosterwijk E, et al. (2004). A phase II trial of chimeric monoclonal antibody WX-G250 for advanced RCC patients. British Journal of Cancer, 90, 985–90.

Bregni M, Dodero A, Peccatori J, et al. (2002). Nonmyeloablative conditioning followed by hematopoietic cell allografting and donor lymphocyte infusions for patients with metastatic renal and breast cancer. Blood, 99, 4234–6.

Bui MH, Seligson D, Han KR, et al. (2003). Carbonic anhydrase IX is an independent predictor of survival in advanced renal clear cell carcinoma: implications for prognosis and therapy. Clinical Cancer Research, 9(2), 802–11.

Childs R, Chernoff A, Contentin N, et al. (2000). Regression of metastatic renal-cell carcinoma after nonmyeloablative allogeneic peripheral-blood stem-cell transplantation. The New England Journal of Medicine, **343(11)**, 750–8.

Childs RW, Clave E, Tisdale J, Plante M, Hensel N and Barrett J (1999). Successful treatment of metastatic renal cell carcinoma with a nonmyeloablative allogeneic peripheral-blood progenitor-cell transplant: evidence for a graft-versus-tumor effect. Journal of Clinical Oncology, **17(7)**, 2044–9.

Clark JI, Atkins MB, Urba WJ, et al. (2003). Adjuvant high-dose bolus IL-2 for patients with high-risk RCC: a cytokine working group randomized trial. Journal of Clinical Oncology, **21**, 3133–40.

Coppin C, Porzsolt F, Awa A, Kumpf J, Coldman A and Wilt T (2005). Immunotherapy for advanced renal cell cancer. Cochrane Database of Systematic Reviews (Online), **1**, CD001425.

Doehn C, Richter A, Theodor RA, et al. (2006). Prolongation of progression-free and overall survival following an adjuvant vaccination with Reniale R in patients with non-metastatic RCC: secondary analysis of a multi-center phase III trial. http://www.Egms.de./en/meetings/dkk2006/06dkk395.shtml. last accessed June 2009.

Escudier B, Farace F, Angevin E, et al. (1994). Immunotherapy with IL2 and Lymphokine-activated natural killer cells: improvement of clinical responses in metastatic renal carcinoma patients previously treated with IL2. European Journal of Cancer, **30A**, 1078–83.

Escudier B, Chevreau C, Lasset C, et al. (1999). Cytokines in metastatic renal cell carcinoma: is it useful to switch to interleukin-2 or interferon after failure of a first treatment? Groupe Francais d'Immunotherape. Journal of Clinical Oncology, **17(7)**, 2039–43.

Escudier B, Eisen T, Stadler WM, et al. (2007). Treatment Approaches in Renal Cancer Global Evaluation Trial (TARGETs): a randomized, double-blind, placebo-controlled phase III trial of sorafenib, an oral multi-kinase inhibitor in advanced renal cell carcinoma. The New England Journal of Medicine, **356(2)**, 125–34.

Escudier B, Pluzanska A, Koralewski P, et al. (2007). Bevacizumab plus interferon alfa-2a for treatment of metastatic renal cell carcinoma: a randomised, double-blind phase III trial. Lancet, **370(9605)**, 2103–11.

Figlin RA, Thompson JA, Bukowski RM, et al. (1999). Multicenter, randomized, phase III trial of CD8(+) tumor-infiltrating lymphocytes in combination with recombinant interleukin-2 in metastatic renal cell carcinoma. Journal of Clinical Oncology, **17(8)**, 2521–9.

Fisher RI, Rosenberg SA and Fyfe G (2000). Long-term survival update for high-dose recombinant interleukin-2 in patients with renal cell carcinoma. The Cancer Journal from Scientific American, **6(Suppl 1)**, S55–7.

Fyfe G, Fisher RI, Rosenberg SA, et al. (1995). Results of treatment of 255 patients with metastatic renal cell carcinoma who received high-dose recombinant interleukin-2 therapy. Journal of Clinical Oncology, **13(3)**, 688–96.

Fyfe GA, Fisher RI, Rosenberg SA, et al. (1996). Long-term response data for 255 patients with metastatic renal cell carcinoma treated with high-dose recombinant interleukin-2 therapy. Journal of Clinical Oncology, 14(8), 2410–11.

Gleave ME, Elihali M, Frader Y, et al. (1998). Interferon gamma-1b compared with placebo in metastatic renal cell carcinoma. The New England Journal of Medicine, 338, 1272–8.

Gore ME (2008). Interferon-α (IFN), interleukin-2 (IL2) and 5-fluorouracil (5FU) vs IFN alone in patients with metastatic renal cell carcinoma (mRCC): Results of the randomised MRC/EORTC RE04 trial. Journal of Clinical Oncology, 26(Suppl), 5039 (abstract).

Gotoh A, Shirakawa T, Hinata N, et al. (2004). Long-term outcome of postoperative IFNalfa adjuvant therapy for non-metastatic RCC. International Journal of Urology, 11, 257–63.

Jocham D, Richter A, Hoffmann L, et al. (2004). Adjuvant autologous renal tumor cell vaccine and risk of tumor progression in patients with RCC after radical nephrectomy: phase III, randomized controlled trial. Lancet, 363, 594–9.

Kugler A, Stuhler G, Walden P, et al. (2000). Regression of human metastatic renal cell carcinoma after vaccination with tumor cell-dendritic cell hybrids. Nature Medicine, 6, 332–6.

Lilleby W and Fossa SD (2005). Chemotherapy in metastatic renal cell cancer. World Journal of Urology, 23, 175–9.

McDermott DF, Regan MM, Clark JI, et al. (2005). Randomized phase III trial of high-dose interleukin-2 versus subcutaneous interleukin-2 and interferon in patients with metastatic renal cell carcinoma. Journal of Clinical Oncology, 23, 133–41.

Messing EM, Manola J, Wilding G, et al. (2003). Eastern Cooperative Oncology Group/Intergroup trial. Phase III study of interferon alfa-NL as adjuvant treatment for resectable renal cell carcinoma: an Eastern Cooperative Oncology Group/Intergroup trial. Journal of Clinical Oncology, 21, 1214–22.

Motzer RJ, Hutson TE, Tomczak P, et al. (2007). Phase III randomized trial of sunitinib malate (SU11248) versus interferon-alfa as first-line systemic therapy for patients with metastatic renal cell carcinoma. The New England Journal of Medicine, 356(2), 115–24.

MRC trial (1999). Interferon-alpha and survival in metastatic renal carcinoma: early results of a randomised controlled trial. Medical Research Council Renal Cancer Collaborators. Lancet, 353(9146), 14–17.

Negrier S, Escudier B, Lasset C, et al. (1998). Recombinant human interleukin-2, recombinant human interferon alfa-2a, or both in metastatic renal-cell carcinoma. Groupe Francais d'Immunotherapie. The New England Journal of Medicine, 338(18), 1272–8.

Negrier S, Escudier B, Gomez F, et al. (2002). Prognostic factors of survival and rapid progression in 782 patients with metastatic renal carcinomas treated by cytokines: a report from the Groupe Francais d'Immunotherapie. Annals of Oncology, 13(9), 1460–8.

Negrier S, Perol D, Ravaud A, et al. (2007). Medroxyprogesterone, interferon alfa-2a, interleukin 2, or combination of both cytokines in patients with metastatic renal carcinoma of intermediate prognosis: results of a randomized controlled trial. *Cancer*, **110(11)**, 2468–77.

Negrier S, Perol D, Ravaud A, et al. (2008). Randomized study of intravenous versus subcutaneous interleukin 2 and interferon alfa in patients with good prognosis metastatic renal cancer. *Clinical Cancer Research*, **14(18)**, 5907–12.

Oliver RT (1998). Are cytokine responses in renal cell cancer the product of placebo effect of treatment or true biotherapy? What trials are needed now? *British Journal of Cancer*, **77**, 1318–20.

Pizzocaro G, Piva L, Colavita M, et al. (2001). Interferon adjuvant to radical nephrectomy in Robson stages II and III RCC: a multicentric randomized study. *Journal of Clinical Oncology*, **19**, 425–31.

Pyrhonen S, Salminen E, Ruutu M, et al. (1999). Prospective randomized trial of interferon alfa-2a plus vinblastine versus vinblastine alone in patients with advanced renal cell cancer. *Journal of Clinical Oncology*, **17(9)**, 2859–67.

Rini BI, Halabi S, Rosenberg JE, et al. (2008). Bevacizumab plus interferon alfa compared with interferon alfa monotherapy in patients with metastatic renal cell carcinoma: CALGB 90206. *Journal of Clinical Oncology*, **26(33)**, 5422–8.

Rosenberg SA, Lotze MT, Muul LM, et al. (1985). Observations on the systemic administration of autologous lymphokine-activated killer cells and recombinant interleukin-2 to patients with metastatic cancer. *The New England Journal of Medicine*, **313**, 1485–92.

Rosenberg SA, Lotze MT, Yang JC, et al. (1989). Experience with the use of high dose interleukin-2 in the treatment of 652 cancer patients. *Annals of Surgery*, **210**, 474–85.

Rosenberg SA, Lotze MT, Yang JC, et al. (1993). Prospective randomized trial of high-dose interleukin-2 alone or in conjunction with lymphokine-activated killer cells for the treatment of patients with advanced cancer. *Journal of the National Cancer Institute*, **85**, 622–32.

Srivastava P (2002). Interaction of heat shock proteins with peptides and antigen presenting cells: chaperoning of the innate and adaptive immune responses. *Annual Review of Immunology*, **20**, 395–425.

Upton MP, Parker RA, Youmans A, McDermott DF and Atkins MB (2005). Histologic predictors of renal cell carcinoma response to interleukin-2-based therapy. *Journal of Immunotherapy*, **28(5)**, 488–95.

Wood C, Bukowski R, Lacombe L, et al. (2008). A multicenter, randomized, Phase 3 trial of a novel, autologous, therapeutic vaccine (vitespen) vs. observation as adjuvant therapy in patients at high risk of recurrence after nephrectomy for renal cell carcinoma. *Lancet*, **372(9633)**, 145–54.

Yagoda A, Abi-Rached B and Petrylak D (1995). Chemotherapy for advanced renal-cell carcinoma: 1983–1993. *Seminars in Oncology*, **22**, 42–60.

Yang JC and Childs R (2006). Immunotherapy for RCC. *Journal of Clinical Oncology*, **24**, 5576–83.

Yang JC, Haworth L, Sherry RM, *et al.* (2003). A randomized trial of bevacizumab, an anti-vascular endothelial growth factor antibody, for metastatic renal cancer. *The New England Journal of Medicine*, **349(5)**, 427–34.

Yang JC, Sherry RM, Steinberg SM, *et al.* (2003). Randomized study of high-dose and low-dose interleukin-2 in patients with metastatic renal cancer. *Journal of Clinical Oncology*, **21(16)**, 3127–32.

Chapter 7

Systemic treatment: targeted therapies

Tanya Dorff and David Quinn

> ### Key points
>
> - The vascular endothelial growth factor (VEGF) pathway is critical for renal cell carcinoma (RCC) survival and metastasis
> - Multitargeted tyrosine kinase inhibitors (TKIs) which inhibit the VEGF pathway prolong time to disease progression and overall survival in advanced RCC
> - The mammalian target of rapamycin (mTOR) is aberrant in a significant number of renal cancers and is a second critical pathway in RCC
> - mTOR inhibitors prolong time to disease progression and overall survival in select groups of patients with RCC
> - Toxicities of VEGF tyrosine kinase and mTOR inhibitors used for RCC therapy require close monitoring, management, and at times dosage modifications.

7.1 Background

Before the development of agents targeting the vascular endothelial growth factor (VEGF) pathway, therapy for renal cell carcinoma (RCC) was limited to immune modulating cytokine therapies, including interferon α (IFN-α) and high-dose interleukin 2 (IL-2). Both sporadic and familial RCC tumours exhibit mutations in or silencing of the von Hippel–Lindau (*VHL*) gene. VHL exerts control over VEGF expression as well as platelet-derived growth factor (PDGF) and other components of the angiogenic pathway. Progress in understanding these important biological factors in RCC resulted in the recognition that inhibition of these pathways could result in apoptosis and necrosis.

Oral multitargeted tyrosine kinase inhibitors (TKIs) were developed to interfere with VEGF signalling and were rationally introduced into clinical trials with RCC patients. In human studies, the majority of metastatic RCC patients benefited from treatment with these VEGF TKIs, experiencing prolonged time to disease progression and improved overall survival, both out of proportion with the low rate of objective responses seen on radiographic imaging. Additional study is ongoing to determine whether there is a role for these agents in the adjuvant or neoadjuvant setting for RCC.

In this chapter, we review the clinical benefits of oral TKIs in the treatment of RCC, as well as practical management of their associated toxicities.

7.2 **Sorafenib**

Sorafenib is an oral multitargeted TKI which inhibits Raf kinase, VEGFR1, 2, and 3, as well as the PDGF receptor, FMS-like tyrosine kinase 3 (Flt-3), c-Kit, and RET. In phase I studies, tumour responses and disease stabilization were noted for several RCC patients, and although no definitive dose–response relationship was noted, more patients receiving ≥200mg twice daily were found to have responses. A dose of 400mg twice daily was selected for phase II studies, although higher doses are certainly tolerable in a subset of patients.

Sorafenib was evaluated in a phase II trial, with predominantly clear cell RCC patients who had experienced disease progression after cytokine therapy, using a randomized discontinuation design with placebo control. This trial documented a significant delay in time to disease progression, from 6 weeks to 24 weeks, as well as a 39% increase in overall survival. Tumour reductions of >25% of tumour volumes by World Health Organization (WHO) criteria were noted in 36% of patients.

The Treatment Approach in Renal Cancer Global Evaluation Trial (TARGET) was an international phase III randomized, placebo-controlled trial that enrolled 903 patients with clear cell RCC who had received at least one prior therapy, predominantly with cytokines. Subjects received sorafenib 400mg twice daily or placebo dosed continuously on each and every day. At the first interim analysis the median progression-free survival, determined by independent review, was 5.5 months for the sorafenib arm compared to 2.8 months for placebo, corresponding to a 56% reduction in the risk of progression (CI 0.35–0.55) (Figure 7.1). Few patients taking sorafenib had responses by RECIST criteria, only 10%; however, a significant majority (77%) had stable disease. Median time to response was 80 days and the median duration of response was 182 days. After the interim data were reviewed showing an approximate doubling of

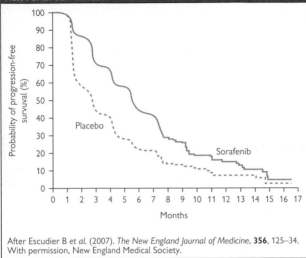

Figure 7.1 Sorafenib vs. placebo TARGET study progression-free survival curves for second-line good- and intermediate-risk renal cell cancer

After Escudier B *et al.* (2007). *The New England Journal of Medicine*, **356**, 125–34. With permission, New England Medical Society.

progression-free survival, the trial was unblinded, and subjects on placebo were allowed to cross over to sorafenib. This diluted the ability to see an overall survival effect in this trial but with censoring of patients crossing over from placebo to sorafenib, a 3.5-month overall survival benefit was seen for sorafenib (*p* = 0.02).

The most frequent side effects of sorafenib include diffuse body rash, diarrhoea, hand–foot skin reaction (HFSR), fatigue, and hypertension (Table 7.1). Overall, 30% of patients experience grade 3 or 4 adverse events but only 10% discontinue treatment for toxicity and only 13% require dose reductions.

Supportive care measures may facilitate tolerance of therapy. Strict monitoring of blood pressure is required, using a home blood pressure monitor if possible, with intervention with standard antihypertensive drugs for a diastolic blood pressure over 90mmHg. Patients should be instructed to apply lanolin-based lotion or ointment to the hands and feet prophylactically to limit HFSR with the addition of urease-based topical agents if hyperkeratosis is prominent. They are also informed about the use of anti-diarrhoeal agents such as loperamide. Dose interruption is an effective means of managing many of these side effects and virtually all patients can be restarted after a break of a week or so.

Table 7.1 Comparison of phase III clinical trial patient populations and results for VEGF tyrosine kinase therapies for RCC

	Sorafenib	Sunitinib	Pazopanib
Median age (range)	58 (19–86)	62 (27–87)	59 (28–85)
Metastatic sites			
>2	57%	85%	55%
Liver	26%	26%	26%
Nephrectomy	94%	91%	100%
Prior systemic therapy	Cytokine-refractory	None	Mixed: none/cytokine refractory
MSKCC risk			
Low	52%	38%	39%
Intermediate	48%	56%	54%
High	0%	6%	3%
RECIST responses			
CR	<1%	2.9%*	0%
PR	10%	31%	32%/29%
SD	74%	48%	
Time to response	80 days		83 days
Duration of response	182 days (36–378)		411 days
PFS	5.5 months	11 months	11.1/7.2 months
Toxicities (grade 3/4)			
Hypertension	4%	12%	4%
Neutropenia	—	12%	1%
Hand/foot syndrome	6%	8%	<1%
Diarrhoea	2%	8%	4%
Fatigue/asthenia	5%	11%	5%

7.3 Sunitinib

Sunitinib is an oral TKI, which inhibits signalling by VEGFR2, PDGFR, Src, Abl, insulin-like growth factor receptor-1, and fibroblast growth factor receptor-1. The drug is classically dosed at 50mg daily, 4 weeks on and 2 weeks off although an alternative regimen of 37.5mg orally daily is also used.

Phase II trials of sunitinib in cytokine-refractory RCC patients identified a response rate of 34–40%, with a time to disease progression of 8.3–8.7 months, and overall survival of 16 months.

A phase III trial compared sunitinib to IFN-α as first-line therapy in metastatic RCC. Objective response rates for sunitinib in this trial were 31%, with progression-free survival of 11 months, both vastly superior to IFN-α ($p < 0.001$) (Figure 7.2). Overall survival data have

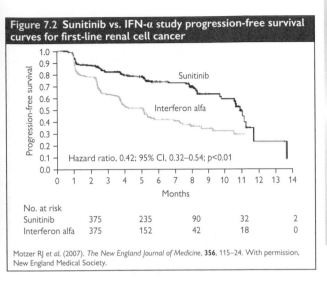

Progression-free survival

Sunitinib

Interferon alfa

Hazard ratio, 0.42; 95% CI, 0.32–0.54; p<0.01

Months

No. at risk

Sunitinib	375	235	90	32	2
Interferon alfa	375	152	42	18	0

Motzer RJ et al. (2007). *The New England Journal of Medicine*, **356**, 115–24. With permission, New England Medical Society.

been presented in abstract form only: the median is 26.4 months for sunitinib and 21.8 months for IFN ($p = 0.051$). With crossover patients censored on switching from IFN-α to sunitinib, statistical significance was reached (hazard ratio 0.81, $p = 0.036$).

The most common grade 3 and 4 toxicities of sunitinib are neutropenia and hypertension (each 12%), fatigue/asthenia (11%), diarrhoea, and hand–foot syndrome (each 8%) (see Table 7.1). In addition to supportive measures such as prophylactic application of lotion to the hands and feet, dose interruptions and reductions are effective in managing these toxicities. Overall, 38% of patients taking sunitinib in the trial required a dose interruption and 32% required a dose reduction.

Other clinically significant toxicities include decline in cardiac left ventricular function and hypothyroidism and routine surveillance for cardiac and thyroid toxicity is recommended with left ventricular ejection fraction assessment, serum thyroid stimulating hormone level and clinical assessment every 3 months.

Overall, quality of life is superior in patients receiving sunitinib compared to those being treated with IFN-α.

7.4 **Axitinib and pazopanib**

Several newer VEGF TKIs are in development, including axitinib and pazopanib.

Axitinib is an oral TKI, which inhibits VEGFR1, VEGFR2, PDGFR-β, and c-KIT. Phase II data in cytokine-refractory metastatic RCC patients revealed a 46% response rate. In patients with progression on sorafenib, 14% responded to axitinib, demonstrating incomplete cross-resistance to these agents.

Phase III data on axitinib are awaited, most specifically a comparison between axitinib and sorafenib in patients failing any standard first-line therapy. This agent is not yet approved for clinical use.

Common side effects of axitinib include hypertension (46%), diarrhoea (27%), fatigue (29%), and nausea (29%).

Pazopanib is an oral TKI, which inhibits VEGFR1, VEGFR2, VEGFR3, PDGFR-α/β, and c-KIT. A randomized discontinuation trial in patients who had received no systemic therapy for RCC revealed a response rate of 35% with an additional 45% of patients achieving disease stability for 12 weeks. Results from a study comparing pazopanib and placebo in treatment-naive and in patients failing first-line therapy, predominantly with cytokine treatment, were reported in mid-2009. Pazopanib demonstrated a doubling of progression-free survival over placebo-treated patients. There was no reported difference in quality of life between pazopanib and placebo.

Common toxicities of pazopanib have included elevation of hepatic transaminases, hypertension, and diarrhoea (see Table 7.1).

7.5 **VEGF TKIs in the perioperative setting**

Given the high level of activity of VEGF TKIs in metastatic RCC, there is active investigation using these agents in the adjuvant and neoadjuvant setting to improve cure rates. A North American Intergroup trial comparing 1 year of treatment with sorafenib or sunitinib to placebo as adjuvant therapy for patients with high-risk localized renal cancer treated with nephrectomy has already accrued over 1,000 patients, with an original target of 1,334 but a recent extension to nearly 2,000 patients. The reason for this was the high rate of drop out of patients due to adverse effects, notably HFSR and fatigue. Preliminary efficacy data may be available from the trial by 2013.

The SORCE trial based in Europe will evaluate 3 years of sorafenib compared to 1 year of sorafenib compared to placebo.

A preliminary report on the use of sorafenib before nephrectomy for T2 and higher localized renal carcinoma reported no excess surgical complications with sorafenib being stopped 24–48hr preoperatively. Specifically, there were no bleeding or wound healing events. All treated patients experienced reduction in tumour volume, ranging from 1% to 54%.

Other studies suggest that sunitinib and other VEGF-targeted agents may be safe and produce tumour reduction in this setting. Additional data are needed to assess the clinical impact of the neoadjuvant approach.

7.6 Vascular endothelial growth factor ligand inhibition: bevacizumab

Bevacizumab, a recombinant human monoclonal antibody against VEGF isomer A, was the first targeted agent to show efficacy in RCC.

In a randomized phase II study, high-dose bevacizumab (10mg/kg IV every 2 weeks) doubled the time to progression compared with placebo in patients with metastatic RCC who had progressed on high-dose IL-2.

Two phase III studies (AVOREN and CALGB 90206) in treatment-naive patients with RCC showed that bevacizumab, when added to IFN-α, doubles progression-free survival and increases response compared to IFN-α alone (Figure 7.3). The addition of bevacizumab to IFN-α in the AVOREN trial improved the PFS (10.2 versus 5.4 months, HR=0.63; p<0.0001) and a trend toward improved OS was observed (p=0.0670), however toxicity is greater with the combination treatment. CALGB trial was of similar design with 732 patients

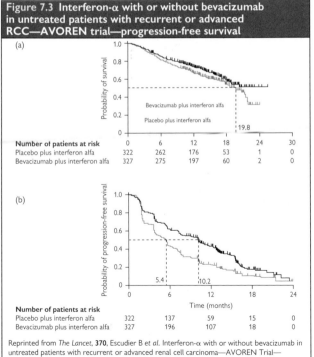

Figure 7.3 Interferon-α with or without bevacizumab in untreated patients with recurrent or advanced RCC—AVOREN trial—progression-free survival

(a)

Probability of survival

Bevacizumab plus interferon alfa

Placebo plus interferon alfa

19.8

Number of patients at risk	0	6	12	18	24	30
Placebo plus interferon alfa	322	262	176	53	1	0
Bevacizumab plus interferon alfa	327	275	197	60	2	0

(b)

Probability of progression-free survival

5.4   10.2

Time (months)

Number of patients at risk					
Placebo plus interferon alfa	322	137	59	15	0
Bevacizumab plus interferon alfa	327	196	107	18	0

Reprinted from *The Lancet*, **370**, Escudier B et al. Interferon-α with or without bevacizumab in untreated patients with recurrent or advanced renal cell carcinoma—AVOREN Trial—progression-free survival, 2103–11. Copyright © 2007, with permission from Elseiver.

recruited. Although the OS has not yet been reached, median PFS was better in patients receiving bevacizumab plus IFN-α 8.5 months versus 5.2 months (HR=0.71, p< .0001). There was no overall survival advantage for the addition of bevacizumab, potentially because of the effect of other drugs used after patients progressed in the IFN-α arm. The addition of bevacizumab increased adverse effects including hypertension, proteinuria, fatigue, and diarrhoea.

7.7 Mammalian target of rapamycin (mTOR) inhibitors: temsirolimus and everolimus

mTOR signalling induces the expression of HIF and other angiogenic proteins and drives cell cycling, making it a rational target in renal cell cancer. Temsirolimus and everolimus are derivatives of rapamycin which bind to an intracellular protein, FKBP-12, forming a complex that inhibits the mTOR serine-threonine kinase.

A phase II study of temsirolimus found no benefit to dosing above 25mg per week. In this study, the observation was made that patients with poor-risk Memorial Sloan-Kettering (MSK) criteria at entry did better than expected. Analysis of RCC from poor-risk patients demonstrated a number of molecular factors in the mTOR pathway that correlated with longer disease control.

A phase III study was undertaken in poor-risk and selected intermediate-risk RCC, with temsirolimus, IFN-α, or a combination of the two drugs (Figure 7.4). Temsirolimus provided superior overall

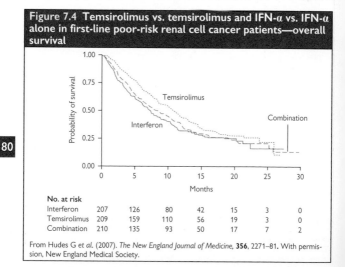

Figure 7.4 Temsirolimus vs. temsirolimus and IFN-α vs. IFN-α alone in first-line poor-risk renal cell cancer patients—overall survival

No. at risk

	0	5	10	15	20	25	30
Interferon	207	126	80	42	15	3	0
Temsirolimus	209	159	110	56	19	3	0
Combination	210	135	93	50	17	7	2

From Hudes G et al. (2007). *The New England Journal of Medicine*, **356**, 2271–81. With permission, New England Medical Society.

survival by 3.5 months compared to IFN-α. Benefit from the temsi-rolimus appeared to be limited to patients who were MSK poor risk, less than 65 and who had non-clear elements within their RCC.

The RECORD-1 trial enrolled 410 patients who had failed one or both of the approved VEGF TKIs, sorafenib, and/or sunitinib, with a 2:1 ratio of randomization of patients to everolimus over placebo (Figure 7.5). At interim analysis, the trial was halted because the median PFS in everolimus was 4.9 months compared to 1.9 months in the placebo group (hazard ratio 0.33).

Everolimus is dosed at 10mg orally (PO) daily, but no maximum tolerated dose was reached in early phase studies.

The most common toxicities with mTOR inhibitors are hyperlipi-daemia (especially triglycerides), stomatitis, rash, nausea, diarrhoea, and hyperglycaemia. mTOR inhibitors may also predispose to activa-tion or development of invasive fungal infections such as pulmonary aspergillosis due to immunosuppressive effects. Some patients de-velop non-infectious pneumonitis on mTOR inhibitors, which is often minimally symptomatic and responds to the addition of low-dose oral corticosteroids. Patients who are symptomatic with pneumonitis should stop the drug and be rapidly evaluated for infection with bronchoalveolar lavage.

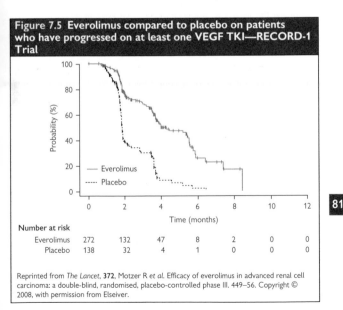

Figure 7.5 Everolimus compared to placebo on patients who have progressed on at least one VEGF TKI—RECORD-1 Trial

Number at risk

Everolimus	272	132	47	8	2	0	0
Placebo	138	32	4	1	0	0	0

Reprinted from *The Lancet*, **372**, Motzer R et al. Efficacy of everolimus in advanced renal cell carcinoma: a double-blind, randomised, placebo-controlled phase III. 449–56. Copyright © 2008, with permission from Elseiver.

7.8 **Additional management questions for targeted therapy in RCC**

Optimal dosing of VEGF pathway modulators and mTOR inhibitors is an important question. Although the sorafenib dose of 400mg twice daily is well tolerated, investigators are asking whether higher response rates or improved survival might be achieved by escalating the dose in individuals who can tolerate it. With sunitinib, the question is whether a continuous dosing strategy with a lower daily dose or a shorter on/off cycle length can yield equivalent or superior results compared to the current schedule of 4 weeks on, 2 weeks off. The advantage to a continuous dosing schedule is less fluctuation in certain side effects such as hypertension but at the cost of the loss of a break from other side effects such as diarrhoea and fatigue, which is afforded by the intermittent schedule.

Bevacizumab is used at doses approximating 5mg/kg each week, with regimens generally using 10mg/kg every 2 weeks or 15mg/kg every 3 weeks. Dosing is empiric, although a study at National Cancer Institute (NCI) has demonstrated longer time to progression with this higher dose regimen compared to lower doses or placebo. In other cancers, lower doses of bevacizumab are being evaluated compared to the higher doses described earlier.

Both mTOR inhibitors are given as a fixed or 'flat' dose regardless of body weight or other factors. Temsirolimus is given at a dose of 25mg intravenously over 30 mins every week, based on phase II and III data. Everolimus is given as a fixed dose of 10mg/day orally based on a series of preclinical and phase I clinical studies that showed optimal cancer cell apoptosis at that dose.

Several ongoing studies will ask the question of whether there is a preferred **sequence order** for the VEGF TKIs or mTOR inhibitors. Retrospective series have documented responses in RCC patients treated with either sorafenib after sunitinib, or vice versa, regardless of degree of response to the first therapy. This question can only be answered in a phase III study and a formal sequencing study of sorafenib and sunitinib has commenced in Europe.

Another area of active investigation is whether combination therapy will be superior to single-agent or sequential single-agent treatment in RCC. To date, there has been more interest in vertical combination (i.e., VEGF ligand inhibitor plus VEGF receptor TKI or mTOR inhibitor plus TKI) rather than horizontal combinations (i.e., TKI plus TKI). The experience with sunitinib in combination with bevacizumab, a monoclonal antibody that targets VEGF and has activity in RCC, demonstrated initial acceptable toxicity at full doses of each agent through early cycles of treatment only to produce renal failure, microangiopathic haemolytic anaemia and reversible leukoencephalopathy in several patients.

Sorafenib has been successfully combined with bevacizumab, though only after significant dose reduction of both agents, albeit with a relatively high tumour response. This benefit was at the cost of severe hypertension and HFS. Combinations of either sunitinib or sorafenib with temsirolimus, an inhibitor of mTOR which is approved for RCC, require significant dose reductions in the VEGF TKI component; data on efficacy are awaited.

The ongoing ECOG E2804 'BeST' (bevacizumab, sorafenib, temsirolimus) study will prospectively compare bevacizumab/temsirolimus, bevacizumab/sorafenib, and sorafenib/temsirolimus combinations.

References and further reading

Brugarolas J (2009). Molecular pathways and targeted therapies for renal cell carcinoma. *ASCO EDUCATIONAL BOOK*, **2009**, 710–15.

Escudier B, Eisen T, Stadler WM, et al. (2007). Sorafenib in advanced clear-cell renal-cell carcinoma. *The New England Journal of Medicine*, **356**, 125–34.

Escudier B, Pluzanska A, Koralewski P, et al. (2007). Bevacizumab plus interferon alfa-2a for treatment of metastatic renal cell carcinoma: a randomised, double-blind phase III trial. *Lancet*, **370**, 2103–11.

Heath VL and Bicknell R (2009). Anticancer strategies involving the vasculature. *Nature Reviews Clinical Oncology*, **6**, 395–404.

Hudes G, Carducci M, Tomczak P, et al. (2007). Temsirolimus, interferon alfa, or both for advanced renal-cell carcinoma. *The New England Journal of Medicine*, **356**, 2271–81.

Motzer RJ, Hutson TE, Tomczak P, et al. (2007). Sunitinib versus interferon alfa in metastatic renal-cell carcinoma. *The New England Journal of Medicine*, **356**, 115–24.

Motzer RJ, Escudier B, Oudard S, et al. (2008). Efficacy of everolimus in advanced renal cell carcinoma: a double-blind, randomised, placebo-controlled phase III trial. *Lancet*, **372**, 449–56.

Ratain MJ, Eisen T, Stadler WM, et al. (2006). Phase II placebo-controlled randomized discontinuation trial of sorafenib in patients with metastatic renal cell carcinoma. *Journal of Clinical Oncology*, **24**, 2505–12.

Rini BI and Small EJ (2005). Biology and clinical development of vascular endothelial growth factor-targeted therapy in renal cell carcinoma. *Journal of Clinical Oncology*, **23**, 1028–43.

Rini BI, Tamaskar I, Shaheen P, et al. (2007). Hypothyroidism in patients with metastatic renal cell carcinoma treated with sunitinib. *Journal of the National Cancer Institute*, **99**, 81–3.

Rini BI, Halabi S, Rosenberg JE, et al. (2008). Bevacizumab plus interferon alfa compared with interferon alfa monotherapy in patients with metastatic renal cell carcinoma: CALGB 90206. *Journal of Clinical Oncology*, **26**, 5422–8.

Rixe O, Bukowski RM, Michaelson MD, *et al.* (2007). Axitinib treatment in patients with cytokine-refractory metastatic renal-cell cancer: a phase II study. *The Lancet Oncology*, **8**, 975–84.

Telli ML, Witteles RM, Fisher GA and Srinivas S (2008). Cardiotoxicity associated with the cancer therapeutic agent sunitinib malate. *Annals of Oncology.* **19**, 1613–18

Yang JC, Haworth L, Sherry RM, *et al.* (2003). A randomized trial of bevacizumab, an anti-vascular endothelial growth factor antibody, for metastatic renal cancer. *The New England Journal of Medicine*, **349**, 427–34.

Chapter 8

Palliative interventions

Jessica Masterson, Michael J. Fisch, and
Nizar M. Tannir

> **Key points**
> - Inoperable and/or metastatic renal cell carcinoma is
>   clinically challenging
> - Pain from local tumour burden and metastatic disease is
>   the most common prevailing symptom
> - Paraneoplastic and vascular complications are a source
>   of significant morbidity for patients
> - Novel targeted therapies and immunotherapy for
>   advanced disease have unique toxicity profiles
> - Proper assessment and palliative management of pain
>   and symptoms in advanced disease improves the
>   patient's quality of life.

8.1 Introduction

Approximately 25% of patients with renal cell carcinoma (RCC) have
metastatic disease when they are first seen, and approximately 30%
develop recurrence after undergoing nephrectomy for localized
disease. Despite recent advances in the treatment of RCC, many
patients face a significant disease burden. For patients with advanced
disease, a comprehensive care plan includes interventions that may
alter the disease course and those that aim to alleviate symptom
burden and suffering. The emphasis placed on each of these aspects
of care should be individualized according to the patient's goals. Pain
and symptom management are clinically relevant at all stages of renal
cancer; after disease progression, this often becomes the primary
focus.

This chapter outlines the most frequent symptoms and clinical
challenges encountered by patients with locally advanced and
metastatic RCC. Supportive measures and treatment options are
discussed.

8.2 **Pain management**

Pain is the most commonly reported symptom in patients with cancer. Up to 90% of patients with advanced RCC will experience daily pain at some point in their disease course. Effective pain management begins with a thorough history-taking and physical examination to accurately assess pain character, location, and intensity. Various validated pain scales may be used for both initial assessment and treatment response. In addition, further imaging and laboratory studies may provide additional diagnostic information to guide total pain management plans. In the assessment of total pain, it is important to remember that the physical experience of pain is often modulated by psychosocial and spiritual factors. Some patients who have pain will not express it as hurting or soreness or pain but may experience it as fatigue or some other symptoms. Thus, the absence of pain expression does not exclude the possibility that nociception is a relevant issue for a given patient.

8.2.1 **General principles**

Although the pathophysiology of cancer pain is complex and not fully understood, it is helpful to think about pain as having two distinct categories: nociceptive and neuropathic. Nociceptive pain includes both somatic and visceral pain and is often described as aching or cramping. Neuropathic pain results from injury to nerves and is often experienced as shooting or stabbing discomfort. Regardless of the pain's aetiology, the World Health Organization's Pain Ladder and the appropriate titration of opioid medication dosage remains the mainstay of therapy. In the case of neuropathic pain and opioid-resistant pain syndromes, adjunctive medications, including anticonvulsant, anti-inflammatory, and anticholinergic agents, can be used. The use of adjunctive agents not only improves pain control but also in some cases may decrease the amount of opioid required. This reduces dose-limiting side effects such as constipation, sedation, myoclonus, and hyperalgesia.

Individualized opioid pain management plans should include both a long-acting medication to control basal levels of pain and as-needed dosing of breakthrough medication to control pain exacerbations. As a general rule, breakthrough medication dosing is roughly 10–20% of a patient's total daily opioid dose.

Cancer pain that is difficult to manage may be further alleviated by interventional measures such as neuroaxial infusions, neurolytic blocks, and surgical procedures (see the subsequent text).

Ongoing assessment is essential for successful pain management. Careful attention must be paid to preventing and treating common medication side effects such as constipation and sedation. Patients may have fears and misconceptions about initiating narcotic therapy, but patient education and a simple dosing regimen have been shown to improve patient compliance. Figure 8.1 and Table 8.1 outline the stepwise approach and commonly used medications for pain management in the setting of advanced cancer.

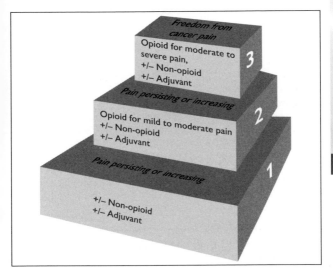

Figure 8.1 WHO pain ladder. Reproduced with permission of the World Health Organization at http://www.who.int/cancer/palliative/painladder/en/. © WHO 2009, last accessed 6 February 2009.

Table 8.1 Commonly used medications for cancer pain	
	Starting doses
Opioids	
Morphine	15–30mg PO q3–4hr
Oxycodone	10mg PO q4–6hr
Hydromorphone	4mg PO q2–3hr
Fentanyl	25µg/hr TD q72hr
Methadone	5mg PO q12hr
Adjuvants	
Ibuprofen	400mg PO q8hr
Gabapentin	300mg PO daily
Carbamazepine	200mg PO twice daily
Amitriptyline	25mg PO daily
PO, orally; TD, transdermally.	

8.2.2 **Interventions for local disease burden**

Control of pain syndromes from tumour burden in the abdominal cavity can also be approached with interventional techniques such as palliative nephrectomy, renal artery embolization, and coeliac plexus nerve block. These interventions are adjunctive to opioid and other pain therapies and usually do not obviate the need for pain medications.

8.2.2.1 Palliative nephrectomy

Palliative surgery for advanced cancer, as in the case of palliative nephrectomy, is aimed at relief of symptoms and improved quality of life. Although it is useful in relieving pain symptoms from tumour burden and obstruction, palliative nephrectomy is most effective in controlling haematuria and certain paraneoplastic syndromes (Table 8.2).

8.2.2.2 Renal artery embolization

In the past, renal artery embolization was used preoperatively to facilitate nephrectomy and stimulate the body's immunological response against metastases. Currently, this procedure is used as a palliative measure in advanced disease, as an alternative to surgery, in patients with compromised performance status to control gross haematuria and flank pain. A post-embolization syndrome of fever, abdominal pain, and nausea may occur 1–3 days after the procedure and resolves within several days.

8.2.2.3 Coeliac plexus nerve block

Neurolytic blocks such as a coeliac plexus block are useful adjuncts to opioids for the control of intractable visceral pain arising from tumour burden in the upper abdominal cavity. Neurolysis is usually achieved with injections of alcohol or phenol. Most patients experience a significant reduction in pain that lasts on average from 6 months to 1 year. This procedure may be repeated as needed for longer term pain control. Complications include local pain, orthostatic hypotension, diarrhoea, and haemorrhage.

Table 8.2 Common paraneoplastic syndromes in RCC
• Hypercalcaemia
• Hyperglycaemia
• Renin secretion
• Stauffer syndrome
• Polyneuromyopathy
• Anaemia
• Erythrocytosis
• Thrombocytosis
• Autoimmune haemolytic anaemia
• Membranous glomerulonephritis
• Dermatitis herpetiformis

8.2.3 **Interventions for metastatic disease**

The most common metastatic sites for RCC are the lungs, lymph nodes, bone, liver, adrenal glands, and brain. Metastases to the bone are the most frequent cause of pain; they are classically lytic in nature and carry both a high risk for fracture and a poor prognosis. Management strategies for refractory pain caused by bone metastases include neuroaxial infusions, radiotherapy, corticosteroids, bisphosphonates, and surgical or radiological procedures (see later).

8.2.3.1 *Neuroaxial infusions*

Neuroaxial infusions involve the administration of opioids and adjunctive analgesics directly into the central nervous system at the level of the spinal cord. Administration of pain medication directly into the epidural or intrathecal space provides effective analgesia at doses lower than those used in oral or parenteral administration. In general, the relative potencies of opioids in the epidural and intrathecal spaces are 10-fold and 100-fold those of equal intravenous doses. This allows for a more favourable side-effect profile in cases of refractory pain (such as that caused by bone metastases), which often require high doses of opioids. Delivery of neuroaxial medications may be intermittent and/or continuous and can be controlled by an implantable or external pump. Device complications include infection, catheter tip migration, and granuloma.

8.2.3.2 *Radiotherapy*

Traditional radiotherapy for bone metastases can be an effective palliative measure for bone pain that is refractory to medications. Relief is often experienced within the first few treatments and reaches its maximum effectiveness after several weeks. Although radiation doses are often fractionated to avoid long-term side effects, patients with short-life expectancy can be treated with a single high-dose fraction. Stereotactic radiosurgery is a novel approach to treat a solitary vertebral metastasis. Fatigue is the most prevalent side effect of radiotherapy.

8.2.3.3 *Corticosteroids*

Corticosteroids play a significant role in the palliation of symptoms in patients with cancer. They are used to help control nausea, increase appetite, improve fatigue, and alleviate malignant bowel obstruction. In the case of bone pain, steroids act as an adjuvant measure to reduce tumour-associated oedema and inflammation and consequently to reduce pain. Low doses of dexamethasone (e.g., 2–4mg twice daily) are often sufficient to provide clinical benefit with an acceptable toxicity profile. Gastrointestinal prophylaxis with a proton-pump inhibitor can reduce the risk of dyspepsia and bleeding associated with chronic steroid use. Careful attention should be paid in patients with pre-existing diabetes, however, because steroids exacerbate hyperglycaemia.

8.2.3.4 Bisphosphonates

Bisphosphonates inhibit the release of calcium from bone by inhibiting the activity of osteoclasts; they are indicated in the treatment of malignancy-associated hypercalcaemia. In the case of bone metastases in RCC, bisphosphonates such as zoledronic acid have been shown to alleviate pain and reduce the incidence of skeletal-related events (e.g., pathological fracture) by up to 61%. Typically, a short intravenous infusion is given monthly, and pain reduction may be experienced after administration of just one dose. The dosing of bisphosphonates must be adjusted according to creatinine clearance rate. Because a rare but serious complication of bisphosphonate therapy is the development of osteonecrosis of the jaw, attention to dental hygiene is critical before therapy begins. The optimal duration of therapy is as yet unknown.

8.2.3.5 Surgical and radiological procedures

Embolization using particles is an important initial step in controlling severe haemoptysis secondary to metastasis to the lungs or gastrointestinal bleeding secondary to metastases to the stomach or small bowel.

Embolization, radiofrequency ablation, and cryoablation are effective interventions for palliating pain from bone metastases at certain sites, such as the ribs, pelvic bones, and scapulae. For patients with symptomatic or threatening metastases in weight-bearing bone, including the spine, embolization followed by tumour resection is an option when their life expectancy is at least 3 months.

In patients with vertebral compression fractures, kyphoplasty and vertebroplasty may be used to optimize pain control. These two complementary reconstructive techniques aim to restore the integrity of collapsed vertebral bodies, thus improving analgesia. Kyphoplasty involves the placement of a balloon into the damaged vertebral body and using its inflation and deflation to create an open, accessible cavity. The cavity that is formed is then filled by injecting cement, usually polymethylmethacrylate, in the process of vertebroplasty. These relatively low-risk procedures are often performed percutaneously on an outpatient basis. Rare but serious complications include nerve root compression and pulmonary embolism.

8.3 **Paraneoplastic syndromes**

The term paraneoplastic syndrome refers to a collection of signs and symptoms that are caused by various substances produced by tumour cells or by the body's reaction to the tumour. In some cases, the presence of a paraneoplastic syndrome is the initial clue to the diagnosis of cancer. In patients with RCC, a wide spectrum of syndromes exists (Table 8.2). Although most of these syndromes are relatively rare, the three most common are hypercalcaemia, anaemia, and anorexia–cachexia.

8.3.1 **Hypercalcaemia**

Hypercalcaemia occurs in up to 16% of patients with RCC. In most cases, the production of the parahormone parathyroid-related protein is the underlying aetiology. Symptomatic hypercalcaemia may lead to changes in mental status ranging from lethargy to agitation, nausea and vomiting, constipation, and dehydration. Treatment consists of volume expansion and administration of diuretics and bisphosphonates. Commonly used bisphosphonate regimens include 90mg of pamidronate given over 4–6hr and 4mg of zoledronate given over 15min. Hypercalcaemia of malignancy that is refractory to such measures is a poor prognostic sign, associated with a median survival time of only 35 days. Therefore, depending on the goals of care, it may or may not be appropriate to treat hypercalcaemia.

8.3.2 **Anaemia**

Anaemia is a common manifestation of RCC, with up to 40% of patients having anaemia at the time of diagnosis. In metastatic RCC, this figure can be as high as 90%. Although the anaemia associated with RCC is generally that of chronic disease, additional factors such as bleeding, erythropoietin suppression, and autoimmune haemolytic anaemia may contribute to low haemoglobin levels. Common symptoms include fatigue and dyspnoea on exertion. For symptomatic anaemia, red blood cell transfusions may be appropriate. In addition, low doses of opioids (e.g., 15mg morphine sulphate PO) may be used to reduce the subjective feelings of dyspnoea in select patients. Of note, up to 8% of patients with RCC can have erythrocytosis, thought to be due to direct production of erythropoietin by the tumour as well as a response to local tissue hypoxia from tumour burden.

8.3.3 **Anorexia–cachexia**

Anorexia–cachexia is a wasting syndrome characterized by the loss of muscle and fat due to an aberrant host response to various chronic illnesses. In patients with RCC, this syndrome is seen in up to 40% of patients. In contrast to starvation, in which a host can adapt metabolically to decreased oral intake by conserving lean muscle mass, patients with the anorexia–cachexia syndrome lose muscle mass very early. Metabolic contributors to this syndrome include chronic inflammatory mediators (elevated tumour necrosis factor α and interleukin 6) and neuroendocrine alterations. There is currently no standard treatment for mitigating the biology and clinical problems due to cachexia. Supportive treatments may include the use of appetite stimulants such as megestrol acetate and, in patients with limited survival (<6 weeks), a short course of corticosteroids. Other agents that have been used with some success include the psychotropic medications mirtazapine and olanzapine. Non-pharmacological interventions include nutritional counselling and resistance exercise training.

8.4 **Vascular complications**

A variety of vascular complications occur in patients with RCC owing to the tendency of the tumour to grow and invade vascular structures such as the renal vein, inferior vena cava (IVC), and right atrium. Rarely, the tumour, which is itself highly vascular, may be prone to arteriovenous fistula formation, which can lead to congestive heart failure in severe cases. Table 8.3 outlines the common vascular complications seen in RCC. One of the most common vascular complications is the development of the IVC syndrome.

8.4.1 **IVC syndrome**

The IVC syndrome can occur in up to 10% of patients with RCC as a result of either direct tumour invasion of the vessel or clot formation, both resulting in the obstruction of blood flow. Signs include lower-extremity oedema and tachycardia. Rarely, the pathological process can extend into the hepatic vein, causing Budd-Chiari syndrome. Supportive management strategies include IVC filter placement to prevent pulmonary embolism, although this may itself exacerbate local thrombus, as well as metallic stenting to re-establish blood flow and reduce fluid retention. Therapeutic anticoagulation with low-molecular-weight heparins may be recommended.

8.5 **Toxicity of systemic therapies**

Targeted therapies with sunitinib, sorafenib, bevacizumab plus interferon-α, or temsirolimus have replaced cytokines for the management of patients with advanced RCC. These agents have unique side-effect profiles that require careful attention and early intervention to prevent significant morbidity and debilitation.

Table 8.3 Vascular complications of RCC
• Varicocoele
• Hepatic vein occlusion
• Inferior and/or superior vena cava occlusion
• Pulmonary embolism
• Right atrial thrombus
• Arteriovenous malformations

The main adverse effects of the multi-tyrosine kinase inhibitors sunitinib and sorafenib include fatigue, diarrhoea, rash, hypertension, mucosal irritation, and the hand–foot skin reaction. Fatigue is best managed with good sleep hygiene and the incorporation of appropriate daily exercise. Antidiarrhoeal agents such as loperamide or diphenoxylate and atropine may be used. Patients should also be monitored regularly for hypertension and treated with antihypertensive medications, including beta blockers and angiotensin-converting enzyme inhibitors. The hand–foot skin reaction is characterized by painful blisters and/or calluses on the palms and soles, often accompanied by tingling and desquamation. Supportive treatment includes avoidance of hot water and early initiation of moisturizer use, in combination with the use of cotton gloves and/or socks and gel inserts for enhanced skin protection. Topical agents containing aloe vera, lidocaine, or clobetasol may also be helpful.

Within the first few hours of interferon-α administration, adverse effects such as flu-like symptoms and autonomic instability may occur. These are best managed with non-steroidal anti-inflammatory drugs and haemodynamic support. Fatigue and anorexia are common with chronic use. Other adverse effects include cognitive changes, seizures, and cytopenias. Hypertension, bleeding, impaired wound healing, proteinuria, and clot formation are the most common adverse events associated with the use of bevacizumab. A rare, but serious, complication is gastrointestinal perforation.

Temsirolimus carries a slightly different side-effect profile that includes metabolic syndrome and stomatitis. Monitoring of the fasting glucose concentration is thus recommended for patients given temsirolimus, and dietary modification and the initiation of oral hypoglycaemics are effective initial management strategies. Total cholesterol and triglyceride concentrations should also be monitored, with lipid-lowering medications being started when appropriate. The stomatitis associated with temsirolimus is relatively mild and can be managed with good oral hygiene and pain control.

8.6 **Summary**

Patients with locally advanced and metastatic RCC present a great challenge to urologists and medical oncologists who need to determine the best overall management plan. Regardless of the stage and extent of disease, a comprehensive and multidisciplinary assessment and a plan for symptom management are appropriate and can lead to improved quality of life for the patient. In addition, effective communication with both patients and their families and the use of treatment plans that are in line with individual goals of care are essential components of effective care of patients with advanced RCC.

References and further reading

Bhojani N, Jeldres C, Patard JJ, et al. (2008). Toxicities associated with the administration of sorafenib, sunitinib, and temsirolimus and their management in patients with metastatic renal cell carcinoma. *European Urology*, **53(5)**, 917–30.

Maxwell NJ, Amer NS, Rogers E, Kiely D, Sweeney P and Brady AP (2007). Renal artery embolisation in the palliative treatment of renal carcinoma. *The British Journal of Radiology*, **80(950)**, 96–102.

Papac RJ and Poo-Hwu WJ (1999). Renal cell carcinoma: a paradigm of Lanthanic disease. *American Journal of Clinical Oncology*, **22(3)**, 223–31.

Richel D (2008). Palliative treatment in renal cell cancer. In JJMCH de la Rosette, CN Sternberg and HPA van Poppel, eds. *Renal cell cancer diagnosis and therapy*, pp. 561–5. Springer, London.

Turner JS, Cheung EM, George J and Quinn D (2007). Pain management, supportive and palliative care in patients with renal cell carcinoma. *BJU International*, **99(5 pt B)**, 1305–12.

Chapter 9

Current trials in renal cell carcinoma

Paul Nathan and Anup Vinayan

> **Key points**
>
> - The advent of clinically useful targeted therapies for renal cell carcinoma (RCC) has resulted in a large expansion in clinical trial activity
> - Current trials focus on identifying optimal sequences and combinations of new agents as well as determining whether the new agents are active in the adjuvant setting
> - An understanding of mechanisms of resistance to targeted agents would inform the optimal use of new agents
> - Given the large number of possible combinations and sequences of new therapies that need to be assessed, innovative approaches to clinical trial design need to be considered.

9.1 Introduction

Targeted therapies have transformed treatment options for patients with renal carcinoma. Many questions remain regarding optimal use of the currently available agents and where new agents should be placed in current treatment algorithms. Underlying these clinical questions is the important but as yet unaddressed issue of defining which mechanisms determine resistance to targeted agents. A degree of non-overlapping cross-resistance between targeted agents has already been demonstrated, but a greater understanding will lead to rational design of combinations and sequences of therapeutics.

Current clinical trials are attempting to address the following questions:

- What is the best dose and schedule of administration for the currently available agents?

- Are targeted agents active in the adjuvant setting?
- Are combinations of treatments superior to single agents?
- In which sequences should the new agents be used?
- Are biomarkers identifiable that can predict outcome with targeted agents?
- What other molecular targets are of potential clinical interest?

National Clinical Trials (NCT) numbers are given for all the clinical trials described later. Further details on each study can be found by inputting the trial number at the http://clinicaltrials.gov website.

Innovative approaches to clinical trial design are required to enable an early assessment of the clinical utility of novel therapies in an environment where many new agents are suddenly available.

9.2 **Clinical trial design**

The drug development pathway through phase I, II, and III clinical trials is well established and culminates with large trials comparing new agents with standard management. This paradigm, however, has flaws in a situation where there are many new agents that need to be assessed either alone or in combination in a comparatively uncommon tumour type with limited patient numbers available. Single arm studies can also be confounded by a disease in which the natural history can be highly variable with periods of stability or even regression in the absence of any treatment. Classic end points such as response rate (the amount of tumour shrinkage according to internationally accepted criteria) may also not be the most sensitive way of assessing the clinical activity of classes of drugs which tend to stabilize disease rather than shrink it.

There is, therefore, a requirement for increasing numbers of randomized studies at earlier stages of drug development, principally in the phase II setting. Novel designs such as the randomized discontinuation design have been used with some success in renal cell carcinoma (RCC). Such studies will not replace the need for appropriately powered phase III studies but may enable improved pre-selection of those agents suitable for assessment in phase III studies.

9.3 **Dose and schedule**

The optimal dose and schedule of sorafenib and sunitinib are still open to question.

Sunitinib is used in a discontinuous 4 week on and 2 week off schedule at a starting dose of 50mg. Emerging data with a continuous dosing regime at 37.5mg is reported as having activity. Progression-free survival (PFS) was comparable to that seen with the standard schedule in the second-line setting (8.2 months), although the overall response rate of 19% was lower than that reported with the standard schedule. The relative importance of both peak drug levels and a period without exposure to drug are unknown.

The EFFECT TRIAL (NCT00267748) is a randomized phase II trial which has two stages, the second of which is comparing sunitinib at a continuous regime of 37.5mg versus the standard 50mg 4 weeks on and 2 weeks off schedule (4/2 schedule). The trial will recruit 282 patients overall with metastatic RCC (mRCC) with time to progression as the primary end point. The estimated completion date for measurement of the primary outcome is April 2010.

The standard dose of sorafenib is 400mg BD. In the initial phase I trials of sorafenib, a dose of 600mg BD on a continuous dosing schedule caused dose-limiting toxicities in fewer than one-third of patients. Intra-patient dose escalation is reported to be feasible with high response rates. This is being explored in a multicentre dose escalation study (NCT00618982). This single arm open label phase II trial with response rate as a primary end point escalates dose up to a maximum of 800mg bd if dose-limiting toxicity is not experienced.

Dose escalations are also being investigated within the axitinib versus sorafenib (AXIS) phase III clinical trial.

9.4 Adjuvant treatment

In most parts of the world there is no accepted adjuvant treatment for patients who are at significant risk of recurrence following resection of a primary renal cancer. It is unknown whether targeted therapies are active in this setting. This important question, which could potentially save lives, is being addressed by a number of large randomized phase III clinical trials. Because of the fact that not all patients will relapse, adjuvant studies need to be large in order to have statistical power. Because of the time taken for events to occur, studies also need to run for many years before enough events have occurred to disprove the null hypothesis. Three studies are currently open.

9.4.1 SORCE trial (MRC, UK)

The Medical Research Council SORCE study (NCT00492258) is the largest clinical trial yet conducted in RCC aiming to recruit a total of 1,656 patients. It is a phase III double-blinded study comparing the effect of sorafenib with placebo in patients with resected primary renal carcinoma at high or intermediate risk of relapse as defined by the Mayo score. All histological types of RCC are allowed in the trial. Patients are randomized to one of three arms.

- Arm A: 1 year of sorafenib (400mg BD) followed by 2 years of placebo
- Arm B: 3 years of sorafenib (400mg BD)
- Arm C: 3 years of placebo.

The study, therefore, aims to answer two questions: Does sorafenib confer a disease-free survival benefit and does the length of treatment period influence this? Patients are recruited in a 3:3:2 ratio in groups A, B, and C, respectively. The primary end point of this MRC sponsored trial is disease-free survival. Secondary end points include overall survival, toxicity, and cost effectiveness. SORCE opened recruitment in June 2007 and is planned to continue until August 2012.

9.4.2 **ASSURE trial**

The ASSURE study (NCT00326898) (E2805) is an ECOG sponsored randomized phase III study of adjuvant sunitinib versus placebo and sorafenib versus placebo in patients with resected RCC. Patients with any RCC histology with intermediate-high risk to very high risk disease (pT1b, G3-4, pT2-4, N+) post-radical nephrectomy are included in the trial. The initial total of 1,332 patients to be randomized into three groups with a 1:1:1 ratio has been increased to near 2000 patients due to a high value of treatment withdrawal.

- Sunitinib arm: will receive sunitinib 50mg OD on 4/2 week schedule + placebo for sorafenib
- Sorafenib arm: will receive sorafenib 400mg BD for 6 week + placebo for sunitinib
- Placebo arm: will receive placebo for both sunitinib and sorafenib.

The study treatment period is for 1 year and the primary end point is disease-free survival. Secondary end points are overall survival and toxicity. The study has recruited well.

9.4.3 **S-TRAC trial**

S-TRAC (NCT00375674) is an adjuvant 290 patient phase III randomized study of subjects at high risk of relapse following nephrectomy. Patients are randomized to either placebo or sunitinib 50mg OD in the 4/2 week schedule for a 1-year period. Only those with predominantly clear cell histology are eligible. The primary end point is disease-free survival and secondary end points are overall survival and toxicity.

9.5 **Combination or single agent treatment?**

Combination treatments are attractive where there is true synergy and where there may be slower generation of antitumour resistance due to synchronous therapeutic effects upon multiple pathways.

However, combination therapies that are merely additive are unlikely to provide any advantage over sequential treatment and are more likely to expose the patient to excessive toxicities. In addition, exposure to active drugs early in the course of disease may hasten the generation of resistance and reduce future therapeutic options. The health economic implications of combination treatments also need to be considered.

Five main categories of systemic agents are available with activity against RCC:

1. multitargeted kinase inhibitors (TKIs) (e.g., sunitinib, sorafenib, pazopanib, and axitinib; pazopanib is licensed in Europe and will soon be marketed, while axitinib is not yet licensed in Europe);

2. pure vascular endothelial growth factor (VEGF) ligand binders (e.g., bevacizumab, VEGF trap);

3. mammalian target of rapamycin (mTOR) inhibitors (e.g., temsirolimus and everolimus);

4. immunotherapeutics (e.g., interferon-α [IFN-α]/interleukin-2 [IL-2]); and

5. cytotoxic chemotherapy.

9.5.1 **TKIs + bevacizumab**

Early phase clinical trial data is accumulating regarding combinations between all these categories. Toxicity is proving an issue for many combinations. Combination of TKIs with bevacizumab (effectively vertical blockade through the VEGF pathway) appears to be associated with significant toxicity. Sorafenib and bevacizumab are active in combination although full doses of both drugs are not deliverable. The sunitinib with bevacizumab combination induces a microangiopathic haemolytic anaemia and has been withdrawn from further investigation.

9.5.2 **mTOR inhibition + bevacizumab**

mTOR inhibitors do appear to be combinable at full dose with bevacizumab or the TKIs, and a number of studies are investigating these combinations. It is postulated that the hypoxic stress induced by VEGF blockade may stimulate Akt/PI3/mTOR pathways. There is, therefore, a rationale for combination VEGF/mTOR therapy.

9.5.2.1 *Bevacizumab + temsirolimus vs. bevacizumab + IFN (NCT00631371)*

This randomized 800 patient phase III study compares bevacizumab + temsirolimus with bevacizumab +IFN in advanced RCC. Bevacizumab + IFN is the standard arm and has a licence for the treatment of advanced RCC.

9.5.2.2 Bevacizumab + everolimus vs. bevacizumab + IFN (NCT00719264)

The combination of everolimus with bevacizumab is being evaluated in a similarly designed randomized phase II study (360 patients).

9.5.2.3 BEST study

The BEST study (NCT00378703) is an ECOG 360 patient 4-arm randomized phase II trial comparing three combination experimental arms against single agent bevacizumab. The combinations of bevacizumab + temsirolimus, bevacizumab + sorafenib, and temsirolimus + sorafenib are all being evaluated.

9.5.3 **Interferon-α + TKIs**

The pleiotropic cytokine IFN-α is immunomodulatory, cytotoxic, and anti-angiogenic. It was the standard of care in Europe for advanced RCC for many years and confers a modest survival benefit to a small proportion of patients. The anti-angiogenic activity of low-dose IFN may potentiate other anti-angiogenics. The combination of bevacizumab and IFN significantly improves PFS compared to IFN alone. Sorafenib in combination with low-dose IFN-α is also active although interim results of a small phase II study did not report significantly increased activity compared with sorafenib alone.

The CONCERT study (NCT00678288) is a randomized phase II study in 130 patients comparing sorafenib + IFN versus sorafenib in patients who have failed sunitinib or other TKI therapy. Patients must have tumours with clear cell histology and be in good or intermediate prognostic groups.

9.5.4 **Chemotherapy and TKIs**

RCC is correctly perceived as a chemotherapy resistant tumour. Many clinical trials are ongoing examining the combination of chemotherapy in combination with TKIs or bevacizumab in tumour types other than RCC. However, TKIs may potentiate the activity of chemotherapy to a point where it has a greater role in the management of RCC. No large studies are being performed; however, there is interest in the combination of sunitinib and gemcitabine in poorly differentiated RCC which is being examined in a single arm phase II study (NCT00556049) and the combination of sorafenib with gemcitabine and capecitabine is in a phase Ib/II clinical trial (NCT00121251).

9.6 **Sequencing**

With novel first-line treatment options now available for patients with advanced RCC, attention is focusing on identifying appropriate second-line therapies. Interim analysis of randomized phase III data demonstrates that second-line everolimus following TKI failure is associated with a significant improvement in PFS. There is also a degree of non-overlapping cross-resistance between TKIs, that is, second-line responses can be seen with sunitinib following sorafenib therapy and vice versa.

A number of studies are examining which sequence of targeted agents is most efficacious.

9.6.1 SEQUENTIAL study (NCT00732914)

This randomized phase III trial aims to evaluate whether the efficacy of sorafenib followed by sunitinib is at least as effective as sunitinib followed by sorafenib. Around 540 patients will be randomized to have the following:

a) Sunitinib 50mg OD 4/2 week schedule as a first-line treatment. Once these patients discontinue sunitinib due to PD/toxicity, they will receive sorafenib 400mg BD (as second line).

b) Sorafenib 400mg BD as first line followed by sunitinib 50mg OD 4/2 week schedule (as second line) once they progress on sorafenib.

The primary objective is to evaluate the total PFS from randomization to the progression during the second-line treatment. Secondary objectives include time to progression in first- and second-line treatment, overall survival, disease control rate, safety, and tolerability.

A number of studies are evaluating agents in patients who have progressed on or who did not tolerate first-line sunitinib.

9.6.2 Second-line temsirolimus or sorafenib (NCT00474786)

This study is assessing whether temsirolimus or sorafenib is the best drug to use after failure of sunitinib in mRCC. In this multicentre trial, patients who have progressed on sunitinib will be randomized in a 1:1 basis to receive either temsirolimus 25mg weekly or sorafenib 400mg BD. Each arm will have 220 patients and the investigational drugs will be administered in six weekly cycles. RCC of any histological subtype is included in the study. The subjects will be stratified according to nephrectomy status, duration of sunitinib response, MSKCC prognostic group, and RCC tumour histology. The primary end point of the study will be PFS.

9.6.3 The AXIS trial (NCT00678392)

Axitinib (AG-013736) is a potent second generation TKI inhibiting VEGFR 1, 2, and 3 amongst other kinases. In the phase II trial (NCT00076011), it showed 2 complete and 21 partial responses with an objective response rate of 44.2% (95% CI 30.5–58.7). Median response duration was 23.0 months (20.9–not estimable; range 4.2–29.8). Median time to progression was 15.7 months (8.4–23.4, range 0.03–31.5) and median overall survival was 29.9 months (20.3–not estimable; range 2.4–35.8). The AXIS trial is a phase III randomized control trial comparing axitinib and sorafenib as a second-line treatment in metastatic RCC. A total of 540 RCC patients with mRCC with clear cell histology who have failed their first-line therapy will be randomized to receive either axitinib (starting dose of 5mg BD) or sorafenib (400mg BD). PFS will be the primary outcome measure and secondary outcome measure will include overall survival, response rate, safety, and tolerability.

9.6.4 **New agents in first-line clinical studies**

A number of multitargeted TKIs and mTOR inhibitors are in development by a variety of pharmaceutical companies. Some are being evaluated in advanced RCC.

9.6.4.1 COMPARZ TRIAL (NCT00720941)

This study is being conducted to provide a direct comparison of the efficacy, safety, and tolerability of pazopanib with sunitinib. Pazopanib (GW786034) is a second generation TKI with activity against VEGFR 1, 2, and 3, PDGFR-B, and c-kit.

A total of 876 patients will be randomized in COMPARZ to receive either pazopanib 800mg OD or sunitinib 50mg OD 4/2 week schedule. Primary end point is PFS. Secondary end points include OS, time to response, response rate, and quality of life.

9.6.4.2 The DAST trial (NCT00664326)

The DAST trial is a phase II open label single arm study of a second generation TKI (BAY 73-4506) in metastatic RCC as a first-line treatment. Only clear cell or predominantly clear cell histology and patients with good or intermediate prognosis according to MSKCC criteria are included in this trial. Patients receive BAY 73-4506 160mg OD for 3 weeks of every 4 week cycle. The primary objective is response rate.

9.6.4.3 Cediranib (AZD 2171) (NCT00423332)

This is a phase II double-blinded randomized discontinuation design placebo controlled trial to assess the efficacy and safety profile of cediranib at a starting dose of 45mg OD.

9.6.4.4 The RAPTOR TRIAL (NCT00688753)

This trial evaluates the efficacy of everolimus (RAD001) in first-line metastatic papillary carcinoma of the kidney. This minority histological subtype is frequently excluded from clinical trials of targeted agents. This is a single arm multicentre study with efficacy and safety end points.

9.7 **Surgical studies**

It is unknown whether the new agents have a role before surgery with curative (neoadjuvant) or palliative intent. Cytoreductive nephrectomy provides a survival benefit in patients with advanced disease who go on to receive IFN. The CARMENA study is assessing whether similar benefit is seen with sunitinib. Treating patients with advanced disease and a primary cancer in situ who are then to undergo cytoreductive nephrectomy provides a powerful opportunity to gain an insight into the changes induced in the tumour upon exposure to drug. A number of small-scale studies are therefore underway in which patients undergo pre-treatment biopsies that are then compared with the nephrectomy specimen after a period of drug exposure.

The CARMENA study is a French intergroup trial in which 576 patients with core biopsy proven clear cell RCC and metastatic disease are randomized to undergo nephrectomy or not. All patients will receive sunitinib.

A number of other studies are examining preoperative sunitinib (NCT00480935, NCT00626509, NCT00717587, NCT00715442) or sorafenib (NCT00480389, NCT00405366).

There is a proposed EORTC study comparing sunitinib followed by nephrectomy followed by sunitinib.

9.8 **Summary**

The advent of multiple new therapies with proven activity in RCC has led to a proliferation of clinical trials that are aimed at identifying how the currently available agents may be optimally used. The major themes have been described. There are over 500 trials in RCC currently registered on the NCT database, many of which are evaluating novel therapies and targets in early phase clinical studies. There is, therefore, hope that the recent major advances in the treatment of this refractory disease will be consolidated and improved upon in the near future.

References and further reading

Azad NS, Posadas EM, Kwitkowski VE, et al. (2008). Combination targeted therapy with sorafenib and bevacizumab results in enhanced toxicity and antitumor activity. *Journal of Clinical Oncology*, **26(22)**, 3709–14.

Escudier B, Pluzanska A, Koralewski P, et al. (2007). Bevacizumab plus interferon alfa-2a for treatment of metastatic renal cell carcinoma: a randomised, double-blind phase III trial. *Lancet*, **370(9605)**, 2103–11.

FDA (2008). Microangiopathic Hemolytic Anemia (MAHA) in patients treated with Avastin® (bevacizumab) and sunitinib malate. www.drugs.com last accessed June 2009

Flanigan RC, Mickisch G, Sylvester R, Tangen C, Van Poppel H and Crawford ED (2004). Cytoreductive nephrectomy in patients with metastatic renal cancer: a combined analysis. *Journal of Urology*, **171(3)**, 1071–6.

Ryan CW, Goldman BH, Lara PN Jr, *et al.* (2007). Sorafenib with interferon alfa-2b as first-line treatment of advanced renal carcinoma: a phase II study of the Southwest Oncology Group. *Journal of Clinical Oncology*, **25(22)**, 3296–301.

Tamaskar I, Garcia JA, Elson P, *et al.* (2008). Antitumor effects of sunitinib or sorafenib in patients with metastatic renal cell carcinoma who received prior antiangiogenic therapy. *Journal of Urology*, **179(1)**, 81–6; discussion 86.

Tannir NM, Zurita AJ, Heymach JV, *et al.* (2008). A randomized phase II trial of sorafenib versus sorafenib plus low-dose interferon-alfa: clinical results and biomarker analysis. *Journal of Clinical Oncology* (Meeting Abstracts), **26(15 suppl)**, 5093.

Index